The Social Basis
of Community Care

The
Social Basis
of
Community Care

MARTIN BULMER

*London School of Economics
and Political Science*

London
ALLEN & UNWIN
Boston   Sydney   Wellington

Allen & Unwin, the academic imprint of
Unwin Hyman Ltd
PO Box 18, Park Lane, Hemel Hempstead, Herts HP2 4TE, UK
40 Museum Street, London WC1A 1LU, UK
37/39 Queen Elizabeth Street, London SE1 2QB, UK

Allen & Unwin Inc.,
8 Winchester Place, Winchester, Mass. 01890, USA

Allen & Unwin (Australia) Ltd,
8 Napier Street, North Sydney, NSW 2060, Australia

Allen & Unwin (New Zealand) Ltd in association with the Port
Nicholson Press Ltd,
60 Cambridge Terrace, Wellington, New Zealand

First published in 1987

British Library Cataloguing in Publication Data

Bulmer, Martin
   The social basis of community care.
1. Public welfare – Great Britain
2. Volunteer workers in social service –
Great Britain
I. Title
362.1'0425   HV245

ISBN 0–04–361072–2
ISBN 0–04–361073–0 Pbk

Library of Congress Cataloging-in-Publication Data

Bulmer, Martin
   The social basis of community care.
Bibliography: p.
Includes index.
1. Social service. 2. Social policy. 3. Community
organization. 4. Social service – Great Britain.
5. Great Britain – Social policy. 6. Community organization
– Great Britain. I. Title. II. Title: Community
care.
HV40.B885 1987 361.8'0941 87–988

ISBN 0–04–361072–2 (alk. paper)
ISBN 0–04–361073–0 (pbk. :alk. paper)

Typeset in 10 on 12 pt Bembo by Computerised Typesetting Services
and printed in Great Britain by Billings & Sons, London and Worcester

Contents

Preface

This book is about the relationship between ideas and policy. The policy with which it is concerned is known as 'community care', the support by informal and formal carers of the elderly, the disabled, the mentally ill, the mentally handicapped and other dependent groups in 'the community', who are usually in their own homes, rather than in institutions. The ideas with which this work deals are a mixture of sociological propositions about the nature of modern community life, including personal ties between, in particular, relatives, friends and neighbours, and bowdlerized versions of these ideas which have found their way into the discourse of policy-makers. A central purpose in writing the book is to suggest that, in significant respects, 'community care' policies rest upon fallacious common-sense assumptions which are wrongly presented by policy-makers as sociological truths. As a result there is a vacuum at the heart of care policy which is likely to lead to ineffective or deteriorating provision of services, to the extent that care is transferred to 'the community'. Everyone interested in 'community care', whether as student, practitioner or citizen, needs to aware that this vacuum is being created.

As a policy, 'community care' is of relatively recent origin. Its history is traced in outline in Chapter 1. It is only within the last twenty years that the term has come into extensive use, and even more recently that it has been articulated as a consistent policy. The earliest use of the term was in the area of mental health, as awareness developed of the negative consequences of institutionalizing mental patients in hospitals for long periods. In the United States, and more recently in Britain, policies were instituted to reduce and in some cases close large mental hospitals and mental handicap hospitals, and to discharge the ex-patients into the community, where they would live in hostel-type accommodation or in their own homes and be cared for by a mixture of professional and personal carers, particularly in day centres and by nursing staff on the one hand and by members of their own families on the other.

'Community care' also refers, importantly, to policies aiming to avoid the institutionalization of other dependent groups in the population. In Britain, 95 per cent of the elderly still live in their own homes, and the more frail and immobile (particularly concentrated among the over 75s) are enabled to do so by a mixture of personal care by kin, neighbours and friends and statutory care by district nurses, home helps, social workers, G.P.s and various organized activities such as meals-on-wheels and day centres. Voluntary provision is also an important resource through formal organizations such as Women's Royal Voluntary Service (WRVS) and Help the Aged, and via more informally run neighbourhood care groups. To some extent 'community care' policy merely recognized more explicitly the nature and range of existing provision. 'Informal care' has a pedigree as long as human history. The salience of 'community care' in the 1960s and 1970s stemmed in part from the rapid growth of the personal social services and the perceived need to clarify the boundary between formal and informal provision. There were also, however, moves to plan for it more explicitly, starting with the Seebohm Report on the organization of the personal social services in the late 1960s, and more recently centre-stage in the Barclay Report of 1982 on the roles and tasks of social workers, which recommended a new place for social workers as social care planners integrating formal and informal care. More recently the Audit Commission (1986) has cast a critical eye over the whole field.

One important theme of recent policy discussion has been the need to link formal with informal care in the community, often using the metaphor of 'interweaving'. During the 1980s this has been associated in central government thinking with an enhanced role for the voluntary and private sectors of care (the latter mainly institutional) and with reductions in expenditure on statutory personal social services. Indeed, in September 1984 the Secretary of State for Social Services envisaged a changing role for local authority social service departments as co-ordinators of care provided by voluntary, private and informal carers as well as local government. There have been difficulties in providing flesh for the bones of this new conception, but the fact that it was proposed was indicative of the importance which 'community care' had assumed.

In the health field, mental health and mental handicap policies have focused attention both on professionals as supporters in the community – for example the psychiatric nurse – and on informal carers and their ability to cope with more demanding ex-patients. In the nursing field, the Cumberlege Report (DHSS, 1986) has recently called for a reorientation of nursing services toward care in the community, and the breaking down of barriers and wasteful duplication between, for example, district nurses and health visitors. Here, too, the precise connections within formal care and between formal and informal care are being examined and reformulated.

The ideas with which this book are concerned stem from sociological studies of communities and of urban and rural settlements, and, more generally, of primary groups, personal ties and social networks. The aim is not to provide an exegesis of this literature, but to criticize the use of bowdlerized versions of these ideas in the policy debates over 'community care', to show the divergence between their use in this context and their correct sociological usage, and to pinpoint some of the misapprehensions to which such misuse of the terminology has given rise. The most glaring misuse, discussed in Chapter 2, is the term 'community care' itself and the question of what it actually refers to.

The late Philip Abrams once observed that 'community care' usually meant care by female kin. Discussion of 'community care' necessitates considering the position of women as carers, and the extent to which the provision of care depends upon women's unpaid labour. At the same time, social and demographic trends are reducing the number of women available to provide care, while increasing divorce and remarriage will have as yet unknown effects upon the future care of the elderly by their own families. Although these changes are touched on at several points in the discussion, this work is not a study of the changing position of women or of the family in modern society, both of which are well-treated elsewhere in the literature.

'Community' as a concept invokes images of the family to convey the warmth and intimacy which its bonds are supposed to foster. As will be shown, the term 'community care' appeals to sentiment and postulates a range of supportive ties which may not actually exist in practice, thus putting the burden of care upon particular family members. ('Community care' is used henceforth without inverted commas, but these reservations should be borne in mind.) The appeal to 'informal networks', discussed in Chapter 4, is another case in point, where the anthropological and sociological literature has been misunderstood by those seeking to draw upon it for policy purposes. In one sense, then, this essay might be regarded as a study in *mis*applied social research.

It would be mere academic hubris to claim that policy-makers are unfamiliar with, or ignorant of, social science. Such a fact would be unsurprising. What is more serious is that policy-makers have tended to misconceive the nature of the informal social relationships existing in 'the community', which are portrayed much more accurately in the results of social science research and consequent theoretical reformulation. *The Social Basis of Community Care* seeks to clarify some of these issues in order to enable more realistic policies and practices to be pursued in the future.

The arrangement of the book is as follows. Chapter 1 examines the meaning of 'community care' and 'care', while Chapter 2 draws on the sociological literature on community and urbanism to ask what 'community' means in this context. The third chapter looks briefly at the extent of care undertaken by kin, neighbours and friends, and examines some of the barriers to the provision of such care, both as a result of isolation and loneliness, and as a result of a desire to preserve personal privacy. Chapter 4 takes up the notion of 'informal networks' and asks how applicable these are to the mobilization of informal care. Chapter 5 asks why people care and what the philosophical and sociological bases of doing so are. Chapter 6 considers the obstacles in the the way of 'interweaving' informal and formal care and asks how they might be overcome. The concluding chapter considers future policy issues concerning informal care in the light of the preceding discussion.

This book provides a *tour d'horizon* of the field of community care and seeks to pose challenging questions which, in the author's view, have been insufficiently addressed by policy-makers in this area. It draws on relevant research where appropriate, but does not aim to be a research monograph nor a comprehensive synthesis of existing work, guides to which are available elsewhere (cf. Walker, 1982; Johnson and Cooper, 1984; Parker, 1985; Willmott, 1986a). It seeks to pose questions, answers to many of which are not provided here. Asking the right questions, however, has an important function, particularly in a salient policy area where in the past policies have often not been adequately grounded in sociological reality. Policy-makers have not asked the right questions, and they need to be encouraged to do so.

My interest in these issues began during the academic year 1983–1984, when I prepared with the support of the Joseph Rowntree Memorial Trust an account of the late Philip Abrams's work on neighbours and neighbourhood care, published as *Neighbours: the work of Philip Abrams* (Bulmer, 1986a). The Trust very generously agreed to support a further term's leave of absence from teaching, in the Summer Term 1986, which enabled the present work to be completed. I would like to acknowledge here my debt to the Trustees and to the Trust's Director, Robin Guthrie, for their support for this further period, which forms part of their broader interest in social care research.

My intellectual debts will be evident in the pages that follow, drawing extensively upon and synthesising the work of others in this area. I have been influenced particularly by the writings of Philip Abrams, George W. Brown, Roy Parker, Edward Shils, Robert S. Weiss and Peter Willmott, which have helped to shape the approach taken here. This seeks to integrate the study of sociology with social policy, with a distinct applied slant concerned with practical outcomes as well as broader theoretical questions. For comments which substantially improved the final version I am grateful to Janet Finch, Peter Willmott and my editor, Jane Harris-Matthews. While the book was being prepared Caroline Raffan provided general secretarial support. Valerie Campling typed the manuscript to her usual standard of excellence both in transcribing and in spotting errors and inconsistencies. Responsibility for the text which follows lies with me.

Martin Bulmer
London School of Economics
July, 1986

1

The Policy Context

This book is about some aspects of the idea and practice of community care. It is about ideas concerning social care and how these ideas become transmitted into practical action. John Maynard Keynes observed fifty years ago:

> the ideas of economists and political philosophers, both when they are right and when they are wrong, are more powerful than is usually understood. Indeed the world is ruled by little else. Practical men, who believe themselves to be quite exempt from any intellectual influences, are usually the slaves of some defunct economist. Madmen in authority, who hear voices in the air, are distilling their frenzy from some academic scribbler a few years back. I am sure that the power of vested interests is vastly exaggerated compared with the gradual encroachment of ideas (Keynes, 1936, p. 383).

Keynes was addressing economic policy, but his observations apply with as much, or even more, force to social policy. Ideas about how social provision should be made, how services should be delivered, and the scope for action by government, commercial interests, beneficently minded citizens and private individuals have exercised and do exercise a quite disproportionate influence upon policy and practice. It is true that these are guided also by experience – what has been tried and works usually commends itself to British pragmatism – in the way that, for example, poor law philosophy has been an enduring thread in British social welfare policy. We live in a world of rapid social and economic change, however, in which tried and trusted nostrums may be inadequate to deal with the problems that are faced.

SOCIAL CHANGE AND THE FAMILY

Consider the family as a source of social care. Over the years a good deal of emphasis has been placed upon the role of close kin as potential carers for the elderly and infirm and the physically and mentally handicapped.[1] In the recent past, governments have placed particular emphasis upon the important role which the family plays in social policy (cf. Mount, 1982). Despite the rhetoric, 'community care' often boils down to care by members of the immediate family.

So what are some of the trends in family structure and their implications for its caring capacity? The long-term trend for people to have smaller families is well known, but some of the further implications of this are less well known. Applying demographic trends to an 'average' family, David Eversley has estimated (1982, pp. 255–7) that a hypothetical married couple age 85 and 80 in 1980, married in 1920, would, in 1980, have had forty-two female relatives alive, fourteen of whom would not have been working. By comparison, a married couple age 55 in 1980, married in 1950, would, by the year 2005, when they will have reached the age of 80, have only eleven female relatives alive, only three of whom would not be working. A different measure of dependency is the ratio of persons age 75+ in the population to women age 50–59 (those women most likely to assume the caring role). The change in the likelihood of having an elderly dependent is shown by the change in this ratio from 2.77:1 in 1901 to 1.18:1 in 1976 and 0.86:1 in 1986. By the latter year, there was less than one potential carer in that age group for each elderly person over the age of 75 (Family Policy Studies Centre 1984, p. 17). A different indicator of changes in the family, which has the effect of reducing the availability of female carers, is provided by the married women's economic activity rate, which measures the proportion of married women of working age who are actually in employment as a proportion of all married women of those ages. This has risen between 1921 and 1971 from 9 per cent to 42 per cent. All three sets of figures show that structural change is reducing the probability of family members being available to assume the burden of care which advocates of the family as carers postulate as necessary. The measures are broad and crude ones, but there is no doubt about their general trend.

New ideas – and new policies – have thus been needed to allow for the impact of such changes, as well as to allow for the generally rising level of expectations about standards and scale of social provision. One of the ideas which has achieved prominence in the last quarter of a century has been that of 'community care'. Its use is now ubiquitous in discussions of care of infirm and handicapped members of society. What does the term refer to, and where did it get its appeal? Three instances of the use of the term will be examined, to exemplify its practical impact, before examining the origins and use of the term in policy-making.

THE SEEBOHM REPORT

In the field of social services and social care, the *locus classicus* for the use of the term is the Report of the Committee on Local Authority and Allied Services of 1968, usually known after its Chairman as the Seebohm Report. Seebohm saw the problems which local authority social services departments faced as being the product of underlying social conditions, leading to complexity and intractability in dealing with them. The difficulties which clients of social services faced 'do not arise in a social vacuum; they are, have been or need to be involved in a network of relationships, in social situations. The family and community are seen as the contexts in which problems arise and in which most of them have to be resolved or contained' (Seebohm Report, 1968, p. 44). The main thrust of the report was directed to the administrative reorganization of social services, but a chapter later in the report was devoted to 'the community'. It referred to a wider conception of social service, not directed only to the care of social casualties but to the well-being of the whole community. The community served as both 'the provider as well as the recipient' of social services. The committee did not believe that the small, closely knit rural community of the past could be reproduced in modern urban society. The term 'community' referred both to the physical location and common identity of a group of people belonging to communities of common interest. 'The notion of a community implies the existence of a network of reciprocal social relationships, which among other things ensure mutual aid and give those who experience it a sense of well-being' (Seebohm Report, 1968, p. 147).

In many localities in which clients of social services departments were concentrated, social control was weak through the absence of positive community values. Such common values, attitudes and ways of behaving were fostered by highly integrated and long-established communities. In their absence, in areas such as poorer sections of the inner cities, the personal social services needed to encourage and assist the growth of community identity and mutual aid to combat endemic social problems such as juvenile delinquency, child deprivation and mental illness. It was thought that staff of social services departments should see themselves not as self-contained units but as part of a network of services within the community, concerned with co-ordinating services and mobilizing community resources, particularly volunteers, to meet identified needs. Specific proposals made included fostering community development through neighbourhood groups, supporting innovatory and vigorous voluntary organizations in the locality, and encouraging informal 'good neighbourliness'. A community orientation also involved increasing citizen participation and various suggestions were made to this end. Managers of local area offices in the reorganized social services would have a particular responsibility to relate the offices to the local community.

A community orientation was thus a major feature of the Seebohm Report. The committee saw the potential for drawing upon resources from outside of local government itself, and made a number of recommendations to achieve that objective. Although the Report did not itself use the term 'community care' in so many words, it was concerned with care in, and by, the community and was influential in changing the climate of opinion regarding the responsibilities of social service departments.

PRACTICE IN ONE LOCAL AUTHORITY

A reorganization of local authority social service responsibilities, with the creation of new Social Service departments, followed in

1971. What impact did this have upon policy and practice, and what signs were there of a community orientation a decade later? A set of essays on the experience of one authority, Avon, seeking to develop community-based services, throws light on how ideas and policy had developed since Seebohm (Harbert and Rogers, 1983). In *Community-Based Social Care* the Avon Director of Social Services, Wally Harbert, observed that, when social service departments were created in 1971 in the wake of the Seebohm Report, it quickly became apparent that statutory services were not able to meet all the demands from a sophisticated and articulate public. Self-help groups were useful but had limitations, needing access to skills and financial resources outside the scope of their members. A more community-based approach was therefore developed

> in which social service departments identify needs and go out into the community to locate the skills and other resources required to meet them. The essence of community-based services is that the social services department itself stimulates the growth of voluntary enterprise by seeking out resources in the community that the disadvantaged require and, when necessary, providing training and expert back-up services (Harbert, 1983, p. 3).

The book describes a number of services provided by volunteers in Avon, including family care for the elderly, relief care for handicapped children, stroke rehabilitation and the use of home care associates. It emphasizes the need for volunteers to have at least their expenses met, and to be adequately trained for the tasks which they perform in the locality. Selectivity and targetting in relation to client need is emphasized. Some require prolonged and intensive help whereas others need information and advice.

In addition to statutory and volunteer care, the role of informal care is acknowledged. The long-term decline of the family as a social and economic unit is diagnosed, evident in increased mobility, growing family break-up and the loosening of family ties, with consequences for the care of children in need, the physically and mentally handicapped and the dependent elderly. 'Not only are numbers in these groups increasing, but a changing philosophy away from institutional to community care has placed an unprecedented burden on the community' (Harbert, 1983, p. 5).

The continuing importance, nevertheless, of informal care is evident, focused in the nuclear family and the local neighbourhood.

> The primary task of public and voluntary services is to support the informal care provided by relatives and friends so that the caring relationship continues to meet the pressing needs of the client. Sometimes this support may involve assisting with relatively simple tasks like providing companionship or undertaking domestic chores. At the other extreme it may involve total care to enable relatives to have a break (Harbert, 1983, p. 6).

Informal carers usually lack useful training, which leads people to think that, for example, a frail, elderly person needs professional care by nurses and doctors or by paid staff in a residential institution. This is not so.

> Care, companionship and a willingness to help others is available in great abundance in the community; what we need is the skill and flair to turn that huge potential to the advantage of those who need care. That is the primary task of social service departments (Harbert, 1983, p. 7).

Community-Based Social Care thus offers a number of generalizations about the provision and delivery of social care. It defines community care as care in localities provided by statutory services, volunteers and informal carers working in different ways to support the dependent and the elderly. It defines 'the community' predominantly as the locality, although no very precise reference is apparent. It treats different types of service as complementary to each other, and emphasizes the need to ensure that each is adequately supported. Voluntary care, for example, is not a substitute for statutory care, nor a way of saving money from the hard-pressed budgets of local authority social services. It recognizes the costs that particular types of provision entail. The tone is optimistic throughout. As a description of what one authority was doing in the early 1980s, it stands as a useful marker.

THE BARCLAY REPORT

The roles and tasks of social workers have been a matter of continuing debate in the years since Seebohm, which introduced the concept of 'genericism'. In October 1980 the government asked the National Institute of Social Work (NISW) to inquire into the subject. NISW set up an independent committee, chaired by Peter Barclay, which reported in 1982. This made wide-ranging recommendations about the role of social workers, suggesting a shift from a counselling orientation to one concerned with social care planning. Community social work formed an important part in this strategic shift, and the committee spelt out at some length what community-based practice could achieve. This statement is of some importance on account of the major impact made by the report, although it was not universally acclaimed and indeed included a powerful dissenting report by Robert Pinker.

The Barclay Committee defined 'community' as 'a network or networks of informal relationships between people connected with each other by kinship, common interests, geographical proximity, friendship, occupation, or the giving and receiving of services – or various combinations of these' (Barclay Report, 1982, p. 199). An important feature of community is the capacity of networks of people within it to mobilize individual and collective responses to adversity. Helping and controlling resources available to people in adversity – whether due to old age, parental inadequacy, mental incapacity or physical disability – was what the committee meant by social care. The Report observed that:

> The bulk of social care in England and Wales is provided, not by the statutory or voluntary social services agencies, but by ordinary people who may be linked into informal caring networks in their communities. . . . It is difficult to over-estimate the importance of the social care that members of communities give each other. The majority of people in trouble turn first to their own families for support. If this is lacking or insufficient, the help of wider kin, friends or neighbours becomes a valued resource – first because people we know are often (though by no means always) easier to talk to and confide in than workers in public agencies, secondly because seeking help from our

informal network is, within limits, socially acceptable. Doing so is usually less of a blow to our self-esteem than approaching officialdom (Barclay Report, 1982, pp. 199–200).

The report placed great emphasis on the significance of these informal caring networks, and on the need for formal social services to work in close understanding with them, not in isolation. Social workers needed to find ways of developing partnerships between informal carers (including self-help groups), statutory services and voluntary agencies. 'Sharing social caring is a way both of promoting better care and more care in the community, and of distributing the burden of caring for the disadvantaged more fairly. At present it often falls most heavily upon close relatives' (Barclay Report, 1982, p. 202). In its community orientation, the Barclay committee saw itself as repeating what the Seebohm committee had advocated in the late 1960s, with the difference that, in the early 1980s, reorganization having already taken place, the circumstances were more propitious for a shift in orientation.

Unlike Seebohm, Barclay spelled out what such an approach would involve for the social worker. Most social care is provided not by statutory or voluntary sources but by individual citizens linked in informal caring networks, so the focus of attention of the social worker would have to widen. Individual and family problems would remain the focus of professional attention, but the focus should shift to individuals in the communities or networks of which they form a part. The target should be extended to include those who form, or might form, a social network into which the client is meshed. These networks will vary in size and in what holds them together, but they will need to be taken into account.

Networks may be viewed in one of three ways. Starting with individuals, their links may be traced to others with whom they are in touch and from whom they get informal support. Or the focus could be on the locality or milieu in which an individual lives and the actual or potential links joining people in that setting. Or links may be traced between those sharing common interests, concerns or problems, such as parents of mentally handicapped children, who are not confined to a particular locality or institution. 'Comparing the first with the other two viewpoints may suggest possibilities for enriching individual networks' (Barclay Report, 1982, p. 206). At one point the committee describe social workers as 'upholders of networks', whose task is to 'enable, empower, support and encourage, but not usually to take over from social networks. . . . Clients, relations, neighbours and volunteers become partners with the social worker in developing and providing social care networks' (1982, p. 209).

The Barclay committee was concerned specifically with social work and not with the more broad issue of statutory social services, let alone with the even broader issues of voluntary or informal care. Nevertheless, what the Report has to say about the character of social care and social support is quite generally applicable, and stands as an important statement about the character of community care in the late twentieth century. Whether accepted or not, it provides a benchmark statement of key underlying ideas which helps to understand and interpret the direction taken by policy.

These three examples give some notion of the ideas behind 'community care' and what it has meant in practice. Two of the examples are drawn from influential independent committees advising government. The third shows the range of community-based social care provided by one local authority.

KEY TERMS

'Community Care'

As a first step in understanding how ideas and policies have evolved, it is necessary to look at the terms used in the policy debates, namely 'community care', 'care' and 'community'. The use of words is often an indication of the underlying ideas, capable both of revealing and obscuring the deeper implications of the policies to which they refer. 'Community care' did not originate with Seebohm and Barclay, indeed it was articulated first in relation to the care of the mentally ill. Policies for 'community care' at the present time lie at the confluence of two streams, from the personal social services and from the mental health services. In policy-making the subject has had slightly different connotations, which now flow together as the move to de-institutionalize mentally-ill and mentally-handicapped patients gathers impetus and adds to the dependent minority to be cared for in 'the community'.

As a policy, 'community care' is espoused by politicians of all the main parties, by civil servants, by various professional groups – witness the community physician, the community psychiatric nurse, the community social worker – by voluntary organizations and by local political activists. Community care is widely perceived to be a 'good thing', to be fostered and expanded by appropriate policies. But what does it refer to?

The best starting point for analyzing policy is by looking at official pronouncements by the government department chiefly involved, in this case the Department of Health and Social Security (DHSS). These tend to emphasize the salience of non-institutional care, enabling citizens to lead more normal lives in 'the community'.

> Strengthened primary and community care services will help elderly people to live independently in their own homes; services for those who are mentally ill, including in some cases residential, day care and other support will enable them to keep in touch with their normal lives, and services for mentally handicapped people will enable them to live with their families, or failing that in a supportive local community setting. Such services require the co-operation of neighbourhood and voluntary support, primary health care services and personal social services. (DHSS, 1981a, p. 1)

Some social scientists prefer to emphasize the fact that community care refers predominantly to informal care, particularly by family members. As Philip Abrams put it bluntly, 'the effective bases of community care are kinship, religion and race, not community. . . . Kinship remains the strongest basis of attachment and the most reliable basis of care that we have. This is especially true among women' (Abrams, 1978a, pp. 86–7).

Official Definitions The origins of the term are obscure. In 1961, Richard Titmuss (1968, p. 104) said that he had been unable to discover them. The first official use of the term appears to be in the field of mental illness, when the Royal Commission on Mental Illness and Mental Deficiency (1957) entitled one of the chapters in their report 'The Development of Community Care'. By this they meant the expansion of local authority services. 'Community care', they wrote, covers 'all forms of care (including residential care) which it is appropriate for local health or welfare authorities to provide' (1957, p. 208). One principal aim of the 1959 Mental Health Act, according to the then Minister of Health, Mr Derek Walker-Smith, was to reorientate the mental health services away from institutional care towards care in the community. From then onwards, the term appeared with increasing regularity in official statements. The principles underlying community care included support by a dependent person's own family, friends and neighbours; an emphasis on care in non-institutional settings; the provision of support in the home from statutory services; and preventive measures to prevent readmission to an institution (Walker, 1982, p. 16).

So, in 1977, DHSS defined community care in the mental health field as 'multi-faceted and multi-disciplinary, involving not only those responsible for providing statutory health and social services but also the family, voluntary bodies and, in fact, the whole community itself' (DHSS, 1978, p. 10). In the care of the elderly, 'the primary objective of departmental policies . . . is to enable old people to maintain independent lives in the community for as long as possible. To help achieve this, high priority is being given to the development of domiciliary provision and the encouragement of measures designed to prevent or postpone the need for long-term care in hospital or residential homes' (DHSS, 1978, p. 13). Four years later, the general aims of community care policies were said by the department to be 'to maintain a person's link with family and friends and normal life, and to offer the support that meets his or her particular needs' (DHSS, 1981b, p. 21). The consultative document of the same year, *Care in the Community*, began: 'Most people who need long-term care can and should be looked after in the community. This is what most of them want for themselves and what those responsible for their care believe to be best' (DHSS, 1981a, p. 1).

The White Paper of the same year, *Growing Older*, was equally emphatic:

The primary sources of support and care for elderly people are informal and voluntary. These spring from the personal ties of kinship, friendship and neighbourhood. They are irreplaceable. It is the role of public authorities to sustain and, where necessary, develop – but never to displace – such support and care. Care *in* the community must increasingly mean care *by* the community. (1981c, p. 3)

The White Paper argued that the 'whole community' should be involved. Care of the elderly was a responsibility which should be shared by everyone.

Several elements may be distinguished here. Originally the term referred to care outside of large institutions, and it retains this meaning in the fields of mental illness and mental handicap. There is some inconsistency, because some forms of local hospital or residential care may fall under 'community care', to be contrasted with remote impersonal asylums. The term is thus much used in relation to current policies to de-institutionalize large numbers of mentally ill and mentally handicapped patients (for example, Korman and Glennerster, 1985). A second element is the delivery of various professional services, both to the mentally ill and handicapped and to the physically frail, outside of hospitals or similar institutions. Thus, for example, community nursing means the delivery of health services locally, outside hospitals, by district nurses, health visitors and community psychiatric nurses (Willmott, 1984, p. 23). The Cumberlege Report (DHSS, 1986) on *Neighbourhood Nursing* uses the term 'community nursing' to refer to the work of district nurses, health visitors and school nurses, and calls for a change in orientation in the nursing service away from hospitals toward care in the community. This recognizes the fact that increasingly nursing services are being delivered in clinics, health centres and other more formal settings, as well as in people's own homes.

A third element is the reliance on 'the whole community itself' to provide care, by which is meant in the main care by voluntary and informal care, the latter being provided by family, friends and neighbours. There is increasing policy interest in the scope for reliance on these sources. In 1984 the Secretary of State for Social Services envisaged that local authority social service departments would in time come to play a co-ordinating role in relation to voluntary, informal and commercial care. The question posed was: 'Who does what best and how can they be helped to do it?' Local authorities would co-ordinate care as well as provide it, playing a strategic, enabling role to 'interweave' different types of formal and informal care (Bulmer, 1986c).

Fourthly, in official statements considerable emphasis is placed upon the provision of care as close to normality as possible, that is, in the setting of ordinary life rather than in special institutions. The goal, which is met for the vast majority of the elderly, is to maintain people in their own homes with various support services – in the case of the elderly, home helps, meals on wheels, home nursing, day centres and chiropody, plus many kinds of volunteer and informal support – rather than to institutionalize them.

Multiple Meanings These four elements are a distillation of official policy, across a range of client groups. They suggest a greater degree of consistency than exists in practice. Problems in the use of the term 'community care' lie in the fact that it can mean quite different things. It refers to care outside large hospitals and asylums, but this may take place in local residential institutions *or* in the person's own home. It refers to care in these local settings, but this care may be provided by paid statutory workers, *or* by volunteers, *or* by informal carers, *or* a mixture of two or three of them. It refers to locally-based care, but the geographical area in question may vary from an area as large as a health district for some purposes, down to a street or a few immediate neighbours for other purposes. Kin, where they are involved in care, do not necessarily live locally but may remain in close touch from a further distance by telephone and regular visits. Official usage does not distinguish consistently between these meanings, with the result that the term when used lacks clarity and specificity.

This lack of consistency is an indication of the absence of a clear and consistently applied definition of community care in public policy. 'Despite the reiterated commitments of successive governments and official documents to an, at times, impressive goal, the policy itself has been ambiguous and also insufficient resources have been provided to achieve the goal' (Walker, 1982, p. 19). One indication is the absence of any definition of the term in key legislation. That challenge has simply been avoided. Another has been the tendency to focus on the form rather than the substance of provision, for example, by trying to improve co-ordination between services (between health authorities and local authorities, for instance) rather than putting more resources into domiciliary care. Critics have pointed out that there has been a failure to transfer resources to community care on the scale necessary to implement the policies which are espoused. Thus, between 1974 and 1981, the share of local authority personal social service expenditure allocated to community care as opposed to day care or residential care actually declined slightly, whereas expenditure on the other two categories increased slightly (Walker, 1982, p. 21). Some of these difficulties stem from provision of services targeted upon particular client groups – the mentally ill, the elderly, the physically handicapped, and so on – rather than upon similar provision which would be of benefit for a variety of client groups. Behind this lies the deep seated professional and organizational divide between the health and personal social services which, despite the pieties of joint planning exercises, remains very difficult to bridge and is evident in divergent perceptions of the meaning of community care on both sides of the divide (Webb and Wistow, 1982).

Practitioners also tend to be unaware of the pitfalls into which the language of 'community care' can lead. Conceptual and practical difficulties are glossed over in the account of community-based social care in Avon discussed earlier. 'Community' is treated as synonymous with locality, without recognizing the problems to which this can give rise. While the means of complementing statutory care with volunteer support is spelled out, it is not evaluated. How, for example, is one to decide which services should be provided by the local authority and which by volunteers? How does one evaluate the effectiveness of particular volunteer initiatives, and the impact which they make upon the problem to which they are addressed? To what extent are strategies to extend community care a response to lack of resources in the statutory sector? What scope is there for informal care on the basis of personal ties, given the 'top-down' perspective and the emphasis upon care in the community provided by local authority workers and volunteers?

'Community care' tends to be all things to all men (and women). 'To the politician, "community care" is a useful piece of rhetoric; to the sociologist, it is a stick to beat institutional care with; to the civil servant, it is a cheap alternative to institutional care which can be passed to the local authorities for action – or inaction; to the visionary, it is a dream of the new society in which people really do care; to social service departments, it is a nightmare of heightened public expectations and inadequate resources to meet them' (Jones, Brown and Bradshaw, 1978, p. 114). The term 'community' never seems to be used unfavourably. Just as, in Roberto Unger's words, 'the most obvious thing a doctrine of community tries to do is to determine what sympathetic social relations would look like and thus to describe the political equivalent of love' (quoted in Plant, Lesser and Taylor-Gooby 1980, p. 203), so 'community care' carries overtones of nostalgia, emotion and exhortation which are a particular obstacle to a clear understanding of its meaning.

Richard Titmuss summed up the phenomenon succinctly: 'All kinds of wild and unlovely weeds are changed, by statutory magic and comforting appellation, into the most attractive flowers that bloom not just in the spring but all the year round. . . . Does the everlasting cottage-garden trailer, "Community Care", not conjure up a sense of warmth and human kindness, essentially personal and comforting, as loving as the wild flowers so enchantingly described by Lawrence in *Lady Chatterley's Lover*?' (Titmuss, 1968, p. 104). The gap between rhetoric and the reality of policy is often a very wide one. But though one may deplore the word and its vacuity, 'the term is here to stay – it is far too convenient and carries too many comfortable and compelling images for politicians and policy-makers ever to dispense with it' (Walker, 1986, p. 4).

Care 'In' and 'By' the Community   Can one therefore rescue something from the ambiguity and clarify how discussion of the phenomena which 'community care' embraces can be improved? One useful distinction, first suggested by Michael Bayley in 1973, is between care *in* the community and care *by* the community. Care provided *in* the community includes care in small locally based institutions (such as residential homes, hostels, half-way houses and even small hospitals) in which people are looked after by paid and qualified staff, and care in the client's own home provided by professional, paid workers such as community nurses, chiropodists or home helps. Care provided *by* the community refers to care by families, friends or neighbours, care by more organized groups such as good neighbours, and care by voluntary bodies with a local base. This distinction has now been incorporated in official policy. In the 1981 White Paper on the care of the elderly, it was stated: 'Care *in* the community must increasingly mean care *by* the community' (DHSS, 1981c, p. 3). This distinction has the virtue of making clear the difference between resources fed into the locality from outside and those mobilized from within. It also distinguishes clearly between more formal care provided by paid professionals, either in local institutional settings or a person's own home, and informal care provided by family, friends and neighbours, usually in the home.

Even so, the distinction is not absolutely clear cut. Certain types of formal care, notably the home help service, if provided by local people as employees may bridge the gap between 'in' and 'by' the community, since local people are being used as carers within the statutory system to help other local people whom they may know already or befriend when they start working for them. Similarly, volunteers may stand outside the distinction between 'in' and 'by', since while a voluntary organization may be locally based, it may belong to a large national network, and its members may be of a different social class background and even geographical origin to those who are the recipients of its services. The distinction is also blurred by trends within local authority social service departments to decentralize services down to the local level, part of a wider movement toward decentralization in the delivery of services such as housing and environmental health (cf. Deakin, 1986). At least in intention, such strategies are intended to bring service delivery closer to the people served by them, often by involving local people more directly in care. It remains to be seen whether they achieve this objective. The Dinnington study by Bayley *et al*. (1984) suggested that, while such strategies may foster quite high degrees of inter-professional co-operation, it is more difficult to forge links between statutory carers and the informal caring networks that exist locally.

The Continuum of Formal and Informal Care   'Community care' as a policy cross cuts the actual channels through which care is provided to the dependant. Four different sources are involved:

(1) Statutory care (2) Commercially provided care (3) Voluntary care and (4) Informal care. The first three types of care are more formal and are also more public; the last type is informal and tends to be private. Statutory care is care provided under the aegis of government, usually in Britain through health authorities and local authority social services departments. Commercially provided care is care provided through the market; in Britain notably different forms of residential care for the elderly are supplied on a for-profit basis by individual entrepreneurs. Voluntary care embraces a variety of forms of care provided by volunteers, from highly organized and bureaucratic voluntary associations such as Help The Aged and W.R.V.S. on the one hand to more informal and less organized types of voluntary activity such as 'good neighbour' schemes (cf. Abrams *et al.*, 1981) on the other.

Informal care by family, friends or neighbours is care provided on the basis of affective and particularistic ties which link particular individuals. The basis may be different – common membership of a kinship network, personal affinity between friends, geographical propinquity among neighbours – but in all cases, in contrast to the other three types of care, this is provided on the basis of *personal* ties between individuals as individuals. What the Barclay Report refers to as informal caring networks are constituted on the same basis, and, though the terminology differs, are alternative ways of looking at the same phenomena. The central aim of this book is to elucidate the extent to which personal ties and informal social networks can provide social care and support. To this end, the aspirations of policy will be compared with the realities of actual social relations.

Personal ties are distinctive because they depend upon caring for another as a person first and foremost, not by virtue of the performance of a caring role as an employee, or in pursuit of financial reward, or as a volunteer seeking to help others. To be sure, the performance of one of these three roles does not preclude care on a personal basis: the home help looking after a frail elderly person, the proprietor of a private nursing home, the volunteer delivering meals on wheels may establish quite close personal relationships with some of those whom they care for, so that in time the nature of the relationship is to some extent altered. But the basis of the relationship remains quite different from that of an informal carer – the home help will not provide care if instructed to go to another client instead, and so on – whereas in the case of informal personal ties, care is provided purely on the basis of a personal tie. Other elements may be involved as well – such as reciprocity and obligation – but the reason for care being provided here is the existence of a personal link between the carer and the person cared for (cf. Lewis 1986).

Distinctions of this kind between different types of care have been extended by the idea of a continuum of care, in which different types of care are seen as ranged along a continuum from statutory care at one extreme to informal care at the other. In between lie commercial and voluntary care. Commercial care is close to statutory care, while voluntary care is ranged in the middle of the continuum, itself of varying types.

One issue of central interest is the extent to which different types of care are complementary, and particularly to what extent informal and formal care can be 'interwoven' together. This is considered in detail in Chapter 6, but may be noted here as a major aspect of community care. Community care embraces more than one type of formal care as well as informal care, but how the two may be combined has received relatively little attention. Clarifying the possible combinations is an important aspect of trying to elucidate the concept.

There is also a difference to be noted between passive and active community care. Much of the official writing about community care deals with it as a question of effective service delivery or making local people in need aware of the services which are available to them. Another aspect, however, is 'the cultivation of effective informal caring activities within neighbourhoods by local residents themselves – discovering, unleashing, supporting and relying upon indigenous caring agents and locally-rooted helping networks' (Abrams, 1980, p. 12). Such activities have a more active component, linked as they may be to personal development, community consciousness and to developing local political organization. Neighbourhood care activities in particular may be ways of organizing informal activities on a wider scale and making support available on a wider basis. Much of the official discussion of community care is cast in the passive voice, which needs complementing by the more active as well. The

Seebohm Report alluded to this in discussing citizen participation, but did not go very far in spelling out what forms this might take. The Barclay Report held that the 'principle of partnership between informal caring networks and formal social services organisations entails conferring some share in decision-making on local communities and mutual help and self-help groups' (Barclay Report 1982, p. 214). How this was to be done again was not entirely clear, though there was mention of allowing 'informal carers and communities' a say in how local authority resources were allocated.

Care

'Community care' has been considered at some length. What of the concept of 'care'? How is this used in the policy debates which have gone on in recent years? The term is one which tends to be widely used, its use being treated as unproblematical. The Seebohm Report, for example, does not define it, referring only in general terms to 'knowledge and understanding of social need . . . its complexity and the desirability of meeting it in a comprehensive fashion' (1968, p. 31). There is a tendency in some government policy statements, though not all, to treat care narrowly in terms of the delivery and availability of services to dependents (e.g. SHHD, 1980, p. 12). This is consonant with a passive view of those who receive care, but takes no account of the extent to which they themselves provide self-care or the variety of informal sources upon which they may be able to draw. In discussing 'care', three issues need to be clarified: what is meant by care, who provides the different types of care, and where the burden of care provision falls.

The meaning of care is intuitively fairly obvious, referring to the provision of help, support and protection for vulnerable and dependent members of society. It is not often clear, however, what types of help, support and protection are meant when the term is used. Roy Parker (1981) has made a very useful distinction between care as concern about people on the one hand, and the actual work of looking after more or less dependent people on the other. The two are different, and the latter is better described as 'tending', the more active and face-to-face manifestation of care involving activities such as feeding, washing, lifting, cleaning up the incontinent, protecting and comforting. 'Tending' activities are the 'hard' end of community care, making much greater demands on the carers and posing problems both for the provision of care and its acceptability to the person being cared for. They need to be clearly distinguished from less burdensome forms of care which do not involve actual physical contact with the person being cared for.

By no means all community care, however, involves tending. The care of the frail, elderly, or the mentally ill, for example, may not involve actual physical assistance, but rather visiting, advice and support which enable the person to manage life more easily in a non-institutional setting (usually their own home). This, too, is an important component of the kinds of community care discussed in this book. It has both material and psychological aspects. Material support may take various forms: doing household tasks such as cleaning and washing, doing the shopping, taking or accompanying a person when he or she goes out of the house, managing a person's finances, and contributing financially to his or her living costs. As with physical tending, the degree of support will vary. On the financial side, for example, it may range from just collecting the pension each week from the post office, through negotiation about benefits on the cared-for person's behalf with outside bodies such as the DHSS or the local council to full management of someone else's affairs owing to their own mental incapacity. It can also involve, in the case of family and friends, financial contributions to the support of people who vary in their capacity to manage their own affairs (as already indicated) from total competence to incompetence.

Support also has a psychological dimension. The significance of visiting or telephoning a cared-for person lies not only in seeing that he or she is all right (for example, in the case of an elderly person who has difficulty in walking) but in conveying to such a person the sense that others are concerned about their well-being and wish to contribute to that through social interaction. The importance of such support is evident in the case of those who lack social contacts and live in isolation and loneliness. Isolation and loneliness are discussed further in Chapter 3, and are not the same. A person may be isolated but not lonely, or not isolated and lonely, or neither, or both. These issues loom particularly large in the care and social support of ex-mental patients and the mentally handicapped in the community.

Distinct from physical tending and from support are more general expressions of concern, which may result 'in a charitable donation, in lobbying, in prayer or in feelings of anxiety, sadness or pleasure at what happens to others' (Parker, 1981, p. 17). These, too, are components of 'care', but at a further remove from the person to be cared for. Such concern may lead to the provision of support, but it may not. For example, the involvement of members of the public in cases of child care and child abuse usually remain at the level of general concern, since the tending and support of children is in the hands of the parents and the nuclear family is firmly regarded as part of the private realm (see Chapter 3). It is only in very unusual cases that members of the public report such cases to authorities like social service departments or the National Society for the Prevention of Cruelty to Children (NSPCC). Instances of child abuse are more likely to be detected by professionals such as nurses, doctors or teachers. Yet there is no doubt the public is concerned about the way in which children are treated.

'Care' thus has three components: (1) physical tending, which is the most intimate kind; (2) material and psychological support which does not involve physical contact; and (3) more generalized concern about the welfare of others, which may or may not lead to the other two types of help. Superimposed upon this three-fold distinction is a further distinction between care as labour and care as communal action in the sense defined classically by Max Weber, action with an affective or traditional basis. This takes one into the very difficult area of the values and motivations of carers considered in Chapter 5. Suffice it to note here that while there is variation between statutory, commercial, voluntary and informal forms of care in the components of labour and sense of common fate, this is not as straightforward as it is sometimes presented.

The contrast is often drawn between the paid carer – for example, a GP providing support and arranging tending care for an elderly patient as part of the doctor's job without significant emotional involvement – and the unpaid informal carer – for example, a daughter looking after her mother at home out of a sense of love and duty. Yet the detachment and involvement become mixed, and in the case of unpaid, informal care are always combined. Paid carers may, like nurses and doctors, be professionally trained not to become emotionally involved in their patients' problems, but some degree of involvement is inevitable. As Weber observed, 'every social relationship which goes beyond the pursuit of immediate common ends, which hence lasts for long periods, involves relatively permanent social relationships between the same persons, and these cannot be confined to the technically necessary activities' (1947, p. 137). The home help service is a good case in point. Home helps are employees of local authorities providing material support and sometimes physical tending to housebound and incapacitated people, mostly elderly. Not only do they frequently develop quite strong emotional ties, both positive and negative, with their clients, but the extent to which they (as opposed to district nurses) become involved in physical tending in the course of their work varies widely from authority to authority and is a matter of traditional practice, not formal job definition or role description (J. Bulmer, 1986). In this case, paid care is not simply work.

Nor is informal, unpaid care simply affective or traditional action. It also involves work, in the form of tending or support or both, which is borne by the person providing the care. This important insight has tended to be lost sight of in discussions of informal social care networks and reliance on community ties underpinned by a sense of shared life space and responsibility. All forms of care involve labour, for caring is 'a kind of domestic labour performed on people' (Graham, 1983, p. 27). Physical tending, in particular, may be very arduous, both in intensity and duration, and all tending or support requires physical or mental effort. That this effort has not been adequately recognized in the case of informal care owes much to the fact that it has been carried out predominantly by women, a point returned to below.

Such studies as have been carried out related to people's preferences for the care of the dependent show that for some types of dependency, informal carers are seen as having a major role to play. This is reflected, for example, in elderly people's preference for remaining in their own homes rather than entering institutions as they become more infirm. However, a majority favour the combined use of informal and formal care. A study by West and others in Aberdeen showed that the most preferred care arrangements were community-based professional care: day care centres, day hospitals and sheltered housing.

> There is in general much less preference for care *by* the community than care *in* the community; the public are unwilling to place the major burden of care on informal carers which in practice means the family and women in particular. They are especially unwilling to allocate the major responsibility for care to close kin; the children or siblings of dependent persons. (West, Illsley and Kelman, 1984, p. 294).

If community care is to rely increasingly upon informal carers, it is necessary to be clear what types of care they can provide. Certainly, official pronouncements suggest that the care of those unable to care for themselves should be provided by those closest to them. The family is the first source of support, followed by friends and neighbours. Yet it is important to be clear that different people provide different kinds of care, and there is no easy substitutability between different carers. This issue is considered more fully in later chapters, but some preliminary observations may be made.

In a classic paper on primary group structure, Litwak and Szelenyi (1969) suggested that extended kinship groups, neighbours and friends perform different functions. Kin ties are permanent and most suited to the maintenance of long-term commitments. Face-to-face contacts with neighbours are most suited to time emergencies, territorially based services and activities which require everyday observation to be learned. Friendship ties are most suited to coping with heterogeneity and matters involving continuous fluctuation and variability. Applying this to social care, among informal carers, kin are most appropriate if long-term tending and/or support are needed, neighbours can provide short-term emergency care and some longer-term support which requires rapid reaction and is relatively undemanding, while friends can be relied upon in other situations where an element of choice is the most important feature, such as in maintaining social contacts to reduce isolation.

These different kinds of care cannot obviously be substituted for each other. In particular, tending tasks tend to be regarded as the preserve of close kin and as not suitable for neighbours or friends. If close kin are not available, then statutory carers such as nurses or home helps may be regarded as more suitable alternatives. The same considerations apply to voluntary care, evident in the scope of activities undertaken by neighbourhood care schemes (Abrams *et al.*, 1981; Bulmer, 1986a, Chapters 7–11). Typically, such schemes provide various forms of support – notably visiting in the home and transport within the locality – but do not extend either to the handling of personal finances or to any tending. What sort of care is provided, and who provides it, are thus interlinked.

Another major issue is the question of where the burden of care falls. The matter was summed up most pithily by Philip Abrams, who said community care meant care by female kin. The normative designation of women as carers within the private realm of the family has tended to render the contribution they make invisible or taken for granted, the costs of which have been inadequately assessed in policy debates. These costs include physical strain (the sheer burden which tending can involve, particularly when intense and of long duration), financial loss in terms of earnings foregone, and psychological stress arising from disruption of other close social ties and of life style (cf. EOC, 1982).

> The reason for this lack of recognition is that, like housework, informal caring takes place in the 'private domain' where the sexual division of labour is still imbued with naturalism or functionalism. This view has remained remarkably impervious to the claims of the women's movement that domestic labour bears a striking affinity to work (and arguably *is* work) (Ungerson, 1983, p. 62).

Feminists themselves have underplayed the issue by focusing upon the reproduction of labour power through child care, largely ignoring the work of caring for the sick, the elderly and the handicapped.

These omissions are currently being remedied, and much more attention is being paid to the role of caring as women's work (cf. Finch and Groves, 1983). The assumptions of policy-makers in the present and for the future tend to be that women will fill culturally assigned caring roles. Such assumptions are both descriptive and prescriptive. 'Community care policies, although they are apparently based on the assumption that structures for providing care *already* exist and simply need to be activated, can very easily become policies which create a *moral imperative* to care, imposed upon women to whom nature and chance have assigned a frail or handicapped relative' (Finch and Groves, 1980, p. 503).

These issues related to the caring role of women are becoming increasingly salient, partly as a result of the demographic trends outlined earlier reducing the number of female kin available as carers, partly through greater female involvement in the labour market and partly as a result of increasing attention to these issues by feminists. In a real sense, the social basis of community care rests upon the backs of women, particularly kin, who perform the labour of care (cf. Ungerson, 1987). Social structural realities are implied in the definitions we use. Community care exploits women's unpaid labour. This is an empirical statement, but is also a value built into the gender divisions of modern industrial society. Land and Rose (1985) refer to women's caring work as 'compulsory altruism'. At the same time, structural constraints upon women's roles are being more closely examined, for example, pollution taboos which make it acceptable for women to tend male kin but unacceptable for men to tend women kin or children (with the exception of spouses caring for each other) (Ungerson, 1983b). The wider discussion about whether women play a unique nurturing role is also relevant (cf. Gilligan, 1982; Noddings, 1984) and will be discussed in Chapter 5.

More radical feminists hold that the family is inherently an oppressive institution for women, since it confines them to domestic and caring roles. 'Community care' is a misnomer, since care is not provided by others so much as by female relatives. In this view:

> (t)he 'community' is an ideological *portmanteau* word for a reactionary, conservative ideology that oppresses women by silently confining them to the private sphere without so much as even mentioning them, (Wilson, 1982, p. 55).

Distinctions between the public and private realms are explored further in Chapter 3, but it may be questioned whether this is an adequate summing up of that elusive descriptive and prescriptive term, 'community'.

'Community'

The most problematic term, 'community', has been left until last. When used in the phrase 'community care' there is almost never any attempt to analyze it. The assumption is usually that 'community' refers in some way to the locality in which a person lives, or to local residents as compared with those living within the walls of an institution. Yet a sociological view suggests the need for a much more penetrating analysis to discover both the extent of people's local ties in the contemporary world, and whether such ties, if they exist, can provide the basis of social care. Policy pronouncements treat the term 'community' in a glib fashion, when it in fact requires close scrutiny.

From the outset, the issue is clouded because 'community' carries with it an aura, a sense of goodness. For it is a normative as well as an analytic and descriptive concept. It refers to society as it is but also to social elements which are valued either in the past, the present or prospectively, whether or not they exist. When people talk of community,

> 'this social memory has a geographic referent, the town, but it is clear from the many layers of emotional meaning attached to the word *community* that the word means more than place or local activity. There is an expectation of a special quality of human relationship in a community, and it is this experiential dimension that is crucial to its definition. Community, then, can be defined better as an experience than as a place' (Bender, 1978, p. 6).

When the Seebohm report referred to community as being bound up with a sense of well-being, it was echoing this element in the definition. The same element is present in philosophical concepts such as a 'moral community' or 'community of principle' whose members acknowledge reciprocal rights and duties with respect to one another (Goodin, 1985, p. 158).

'Community' has a definite prescriptive content. It is rarely used negatively:

> Community can be the warmly persuasive word to describe an existing set of relationships, or a warmly persuasive word to describe an alternative set of relationships. What is most important, perhaps, is that unlike all other terms of social

organisation (state, nation, society, etc.) it seems never to be used unfavourably, and never to be given any opposing or distinguishing terms (Williams, 1976, p. 6).

This is very significant for its use in relation to social care, for it carries the implication that association with 'the community' is good and favourable, whatever the context in which it is used. The elision of analytic and prescriptive elements is, however, subtle, so that they are difficult to disentangle. Unlike 'virtue' or 'happiness' or 'rights', the term purports both to analyze and to prescribe.

> Community is founded on man conceived in his wholeness rather than in one or another of the roles, taken separately, that he may hold in a social order. It draws its psychological strength from levels of motivation deeper than those of mere volition or interest. . . . Community is a fusion of feeling and thought, of tradition and commitment, of membership and volition. . . . Its archetype, both historically and symbolically, is the family, and in almost every type of genuine community the nomenclature of the family is prominent (Nisbet, 1966, pp. 47–8).

The line of argument pursued by a body such as the Barclay committee sought to mobilize and draw on activity based on such sentiments to complement and strengthen care provided from formal, statutory sources through wage labour.

The main analytic contribution to understanding 'community' has been made by sociologists. The most common sociological definition used nowadays refers to an aggregate of people who live in a particular geographical area. This area may range in size from a street at one extreme to a town at the other. It is also used by extension to refer on occasion to the nation or even several nations (as in 'The European Community'). Usually, the reference is to a small geographical area, the local community, and this may be defined as consisting of a street, a neighbourhood of a few streets, a section of a town (as in the famous seventy-five 'natural areas' of Chicago – Hunter, 1974) or the whole village or town. The latter use is relatively uncommon for settlements greater than 100,000 population.

Community may also be defined in terms of a sharing of

common interests, regardless of whether those sharing them are in geographical propinquity to each other. Such interests may be as diverse as ethnic origin, religion, politics, occupation, leisure pursuits or sexual propensity, as in 'the Jewish community', 'the occupational community of the police' or 'the gay community' (Willmott, 1984, p. 5). The two types of community are not mutually exclusive – quite small areas may have different interest communities within them – but they tend to point in rather different directions. The use of the term by the Barclay committee, however, tends to blur the distinction between the two.

Viewed analytically, this can be expressed by saying that communal relationships are an end in themselves rather than a means to an end. Their value is intrinsic to their own existence, not serving external purposes. Max Weber, for example, defined a social relationship as

> 'communal' if 'the orientation to action . . . is based on a subjective feeling of the parties, whether affectual or traditional, that they belong together. . . . Communal relationships may rest on various types of affectual, emotional or traditional bases. Examples are a religious brotherhood, an erotic relationship, a relation of personal loyalty, or national community, the *esprit de corps* of a military unit. The type case is most conveniently illustrated by the family' (Weber, 1947, pp. 136–7).

This encompasses all three elements of the definition developed so far, that of geographical propinquity, of sharing interests in common, and of treating relationships established on such a basis as valuable and to be viewed positively. The example of the family underlines the positive connotations which attach to describing relationships as linked to 'the community'.

Sociologists using the concept of 'community' have expressed many reservations about its value, given the breadth of meaning which it has acquired. In a famous article, G. A. Hillery (1955) identified ninety-four different sociological definitions of community and found that all they had in common with each other was that they dealt with people. A. H. Halsey has observed, discussing the Educational Priority and community development programmes (CDP), that the word is of ancient usage but has so many meanings as to be meaningless. 'All attempts to give this concept a precise empirical meaning have failed and certainly in complex societies there is no total social system, that is a social network in which the whole of one's life may be passed, which is also a local territorial unit' (1974, p. 130).

The appeal of the concept in social welfare, specifically to committees such as Seebohm and Barclay, lies in its evocation of an ideal society.

> It contains the persistent residue of a romantic protest against the complexity of modern urban society – the idea of a decentralised world in which neighbours could and should completely satisfy each other's needs and legitimate demands for health, wealth and happiness. There may perhaps even be a special attractiveness in this idea for the administrator of welfare who is simultaneously guilty about his role in the perpetuation of large-scale bureaucracy and at the same time oppressed by the complex technical and human difficulties in the way of pursuing samaritan goals through impersonal means. (Halsey, 1974, p. 130)

Many social scientists have been made acutely uncomfortable by the prescriptive element built into the concept. 'The error which is often made in the definition of concepts of community is what may be referred to as the sin of pronouncement. Students have pronounced upon the traits which they felt should be contained in community and then have proceeded to look at the facts' (Hillery, 1968, p. 4).

Can anything be rescued from this plethora of meanings? It can, and the analysis of local social processes may be advanced, if one refers to the local community and specifies the senses in which one is referring to it. 'Slippery though the notion of community may be, it is certain to continue in general usage, at least for the foreseeable future, whatever efforts are made to abolish it. . . . For the most part we have to accept the word and make it as precise as possible' (Willmott, 1984, p. 7). The two elements that are central to a definition of community in the context of social care are the focus upon local social relations within a geographical area and the sense of belonging which is also entailed in the concept.

Much of the sociological dissatisfaction with the concept has centred on the assumption that spatial and social relations are identical, with the notion that if one draws a line around a village or a sector of a town, the area so designated constitutes a 'community'. A number of urban sociologists have quite rightly pointed out that there is no necessary relationship between spatial location and the existence of social relationships.[2] People's lives and their social networks in complex, urban industrial societies, such as late twentieth century Britain, have become dispersed from the locality for a variety of reasons, owing to greater geographical mobility, rehousing and urban clearance programmes, wider car ownership, changing patterns of retailing and recreation, and the increased bureaucratization and centralization of both public authorities and private enterprises.

A shift has therefore taken place away from treating local social relations as defined *a priori* by the boundaries of the locality, and to asking to what extent the social networks of individuals (in the sense that the Barclay Report used that term) are actually located within a particular locality, and to what extent outside it. Such a network approach is sensitive 'to the particularity of context. It leaves open the question of whether a specific social aggregate is a community or not. It is an empirical question to determine whether a neighbourhood is a community, or how far community penetrates a kin network. . . . [It makes] the researcher sensitive to the social ties available to the urbanite without restricting the interpretation of what is found' (Bender, 1978, p. 123). It avoids the sin of pronouncement. The network approach to community phenomena will be discussed further in Chapter 4. It has already been encountered in the discussion of informal caring networks in the Barclay Report.

The social scientist also needs to conceptualize, adequately and non-prescriptively, the sense of belonging which is clearly part of 'community'. Peter Willmott (1984, pp. 6–7) has suggested that this can be done in terms of three components of the sense of community. One is the degree of interaction between people in a particular locality. The greater this is, the more likely there will be a sense of community. To the extent that interests and values are shared by neighbours and co-residents, a sense of community may develop, even though in other respects people may be in conflict. And to the extent that local people recognize that they live in an identifiable area and feel attachment to it, a sense of community will develop. The first and second of these are fostered by long residence, strong local kinship ties and vigorous local interest groups, and conditioned by the degree of occupational, class or ethnic homogeneity. Shared adversity has also been a powerful factor in the past in underpinning a sense of community (cf. Abrams, 1980). These underlying conditions will be discussed further in later chapters.

Applying these criteria for a definition of community to the term as used in the Seebohm and Barclay Reports, what does one find? Neither, it must be said, are entirely clear what they mean by 'community'. Seebohm explicitly disavowed a definition in terms of the tightly-knit rural community of a golden past, proposing instead one in terms of the existence of a network of reciprocal social relationships which ensured mutual aid and gave those who experienced it a sense of well-being. This definition must be judged unsatifactory. To define 'community' in terms of a sense of well-being is curiously metaphysical, and far removed from the sense of community as defined above. For good reasons, social policy is not framed in terms of seeking to achieve 'happiness' or 'virtue', and defining community in terms of well-being is placing it upon a similar standing, leading to all the same type of difficulties.

The logical objections to incorporating reciprocity and mutual aid into the definition are different, in that it commits the sin of pronouncement. Policy-makers have been concerned with the extent to which informal caring within particular localities exists or may be fostered. Whether it does exist is problematical. Seebohm, on the other hand, appears to reserve 'community' for areas and localities where such well-developed informal networks, and a feeling of belonging, exist. Where they do not, because of population turnover and heterogeneity, a high incidence of deprivation and social problems – as in inner city areas such as North Kensington, Toxteth or Sparkbrook – the task of social services is to try to build and strengthen such community ties. This is to treat what should be problematical as given, or, in social science terms, to treat what should be the dependent variable as part of the original definition.

Seebohm is unclear about what resorting to 'the community' involves. In places in the report family and community are elided, so that it is not clear to what extent reliance is placed on resources outside the kinship network. Where community clearly means more than kinship ties, it is not clear whether the aim is to promote dealing with clients in their broader social context, not just in terms of individual case-work, or whether community is seen as a means of dealing with individual problems. To the extent that it means the latter, this is open not only to the logical objection above but to the empirical objection that it does not fit many of the kinds of people which social service departments deal with as clients. Michael Clarke has pinpointed the fallacy implicit here, the identification of community and its restoration and socially and individually restorative value with the residential neighbourhood. The model with which Seebohm was working was that of reintegrating disadvantaged and deprived people into a local community as a defence against anomie and the dislocation consequent upon a complex division of labour and urbanization.

Yet society has changed markedly. The local neighbourhood is no longer the centre for many of the activities of the more advantaged, including a considerable proportion of the working class. To take but one mundane example, shopping is typically no longer carried out at the local corner shop, but at the supermarket, in the town-centre or at the out-of-town shopping mall, for the three-fifths of the population who have a car, plus some of those who do not.

The advantaged command economic strength and educational skills which permit them to negotiate their way through the world, establishing work, leisure and friendship ties across a relatively wide geographical area, going well beyond the neighbourhood, and participating in a number of different social networks.

The disadvantaged – particularly the unemployed, chronically sick, single parents, the elderly on low incomes and the mentally and physically handicapped – lack such skills and the choice which that confers. 'Security is seen to lie, in so far as there is any, in staying put, where at least some things and some people are known, recognisable and manageable – the postman, the corner shop keeper, the local publican and neighbours' (Clarke, 1982, p. 459). But the local neighbourhood is changing. No longer is it the relatively stable and tightly knit community of the past (an example of which is described in Roberts, 1971). This is true of many working class areas; indeed, Philip Abrams argued that the attributes possessed by such communities in the past were the outcome of adversity and want, which diminished with rising levels of affluence, mobility and choice.

To postulate, as Seebohm did, the reintegration of the disadvantaged into 'highly-integrated and long-established communities' flies in the face of the evidence that such localities are themselves undergoing change, in the direction of less integration and loose-knit and more far-flung networks. Seebohm's model of the restorative effects of social reintegration through the local community is unrealistic. When an inadequate or delinquent individual is put in the 'care of the community', this does not mean that he or she is found a place of residence in a neighbourhood which then provides informal social support. Such individuals are not like strangers coming into a residential community with a strong identity and good mutual co-operation, in particular because they have been categorized as problematic because of their incapacity to respond positively to such opportunities (Clarke, 1982, p. 464). This is particularly true for mentally ill and mentally handicapped patients discharged through hospitals being run-down. A variety of different sources of support are therefore necessary from statutory and voluntary sources to help the disadvantaged cope with reintegration.

While Seebohm paved the way for Barclay, Barclay adopted a rather different, and less prescriptive, definition of community. The criticism which may be made is that his definition is so all-encompassing that the term loses useful meaning. Barclay used 'community' to refer to informal networks between people connected by kinship, common interests, geographical proximity, friendship, occupation or the giving and receiving of services – or these in various combinations (1982, p. 199). Though its primary emphasis is upon the locality, this is not exclusively so and the definition encompasses all sorts of relationships, quasi-groups and groups not normally considered in this connection, such as extended kin groupings, clubs for the pursuit of sports or hobbies, geographically dispersed networks of friends, associations of members of the same occupation such as trade unions, professional associations and learned societies. This definition, which is so broad and refers to so many disparate situations as to be almost totally elusive, is at odds with the assumption made that in every locality there are informal networks which may be tapped even by those who have not previously been part of them.

In his minority report, Robert Pinker observed that the illusion persisted that the concept of community could resolve all policy dilemmas. This was quite erroneous, and in fact no unitary definition of the term was possible.

> It seems that when our policy-makers reach an intellectual impasse they cover their embarrassment with the figleaf of community. It happened in the case of the Seebohm Committee when it failed to discover a specific definition of 'the family' and immediately proceeded to extol the virtues of 'the community' which, for purposes of that committee came to mean everybody and everything. . . . The concept of community can never be sufficiently well defined to serve as a framework for formal and equitable social policies, and consequently policies based on this concept are bound to be inadequate. . . . The idea of community is both intangible and paradoxical. It is intangible because it has not yet been satisfactorily defined in the setting of an industrial society, and paradoxical because historically it has inspired some of the most paternalist philosophies of social welfare and some of the most libertarian ones. (Barclay Report, 1982, pp. 241–2)

The report did break new ground with its emphasis upon the role of informal social networks. This will be considered in more detail in a later chapter, but it should be noted here that the relationship between 'community' and these networks was not satisfactorily resolved. Rather, Barclay sidestepped the problem by defining 'community' in very global terms, embracing informal networks of widely disparate kinds.

In the community mental health field, the term has been used without being clear what it refers to (for a review see Hunter and Riger, 1986). The concept has been attacked for its imprecision. In a critique all the more impressive in that his career was devoted to studies of community mental health, Alexander H. Leighton concludes that 'the word *community* has a false aura of unified meaning . . . it actually refers to a variety of concepts and to numerous exceedingly heterogenous phenomena . . . it encourages lump thinking and miscommunication' (1982, pp. 155–6). He terms 'communityism' policies based upon the concept, using a vague but ideal model and suffused with emotion. In his view, 'communityism builds on sand – that is, it creates projects and programs that are at high risk of faltering and betraying expectations because they stand on false assumptions. . . . Communityism encompasses incomplete and false perceptions about the nature of society' (1982, pp. 208–9).

'Community spirit' is another folk concept which is invoked in discussions about community care. Some, such as Ferdinand Mount, firmly believe that it exists:

> Community spirit is not a chimaera. It is an observable phenomenon. And what you cannot help observing about it is that community spirit is like happiness. It is not an end which may be directly and deliberately planned. It is a fragrance given off by successful social arrangements. And success is not hard to define. It means simply those arrangements which fit in with the wishes and serve the private ends of the individuals concerned. (1982, p. 171)

Like 'communityism', however, such a term is without secure foundation, and may mean so many different things to different people that it is rendered meaningless.

Attempts to elucidate the concept of 'community' ultimately become self-defeating, though a working definition was suggested earlier in terms of the identification of locally based informal social networks together with a sense of belonging. Even the finest definitions only take one so far. The underlying social structures, of which personal ties and informal social networks from a part, need to be more extensively considered, and it is to this task that the next two chapters are devoted.

To summarize, the present chapter has sought to show that the terms 'community care', 'care' and 'community' embody assumptions and hidden meanings which require urgent elucidation if clarity is to be achieved and policy soundly formulated. All three terms have at times been left undefined, or defined so broadly as to be drained of meaning. No doubt some policymakers prefer this to be the case. Given, however, the difficulties which arise in implementing effective community care policies, then appreciating the problematic status of the key terms used in public discussion is the first step towards developing a more realistic view.

NOTES

1　The elderly and infirm and the physically and mentally handicapped (including the mentally ill) are the principal categories of persons needing care considered in this book. The needs of other sections of the population for care should, however, not be lost sight of. Caroline Glendinning, for example, has recently studied formal provision for disabled children (1986). Other groups include certain types of single parent, prisoners' wives and the long-term unemployed.

2　Notably, Herbert Gans suggested (1964) that 'ways of life do not coincide with settlement patterns', Ray Pahl (1966) suggested that 'any attempt to tie patterns of social relationships to a particular geographical milieu is a singularly fruitless exercise', while Margaret Stacey (1969) doubted whether the concept referred to a useful abstraction at all. This wave of scepticism about the relationship between built form and social relationships, and whether 'urban' and 'rural' were useful means of distinguishing forms of social relations was summed up most aptly in Manuel Castells' 1968 article: 'Y-a-t-il une sociologie urbaine?' Criticism of what locality studies explained resonated with more general critiques of urban sociology from a political economy standpoint, such as those of David Harvey (1973) and Manuel Castells (1977). The focus of interest shifted to the regional, national and international levels. Local communities were no longer held to be in command of their own economic and political fate (if they ever were). Thus, what could be explained by studying local social relations *per se* was severely limited.

　　The traces left by this critique of the Simmel-Wirth tradition of urban sociology spread wider. Studies of 'urban villages', within urban areas, showed that people *did* retain attachments and there were small social worlds where something of the *gemeinschaft*-like qualities of an earlier age persisted. The most notable of these were Young and Willmott's study of Bethnal Green in East London (1957) and Herbert Gans's study of an Italian inner area of Boston (1962), but there were others (cf. Suttles, 1968; Fried, 1973; Stack, 1974). Philip Abrams suggested (1978, p. 10) a more radical step: getting rid of the concept of the town.

2

The Sociological Context

Community care involves the provision of care and support both *in* the community and *by* the community, variously from statutory, commercial, voluntary and informal carers, with a particular emphasis upon the latter. Depending upon the client's condition, there is a greater or lesser chance of paid carers being involved. It is perhaps highest for the mentally ill. How is the sociological context in which this care is provided changing, and what more general theories can one use to make sense of trends in this area? It is particularly important to understand how society is changing in order not to promulgate policies entailing unrealistic or false expectations. This chapter and the next explore theories and evidence about informal social relationships to throw light upon some of the conditions out of which informal social care can develop.

This involves both a brief excursion into sociological theories of social change, and a more extended consideration of the 'decline of community' thesis and trends toward privatization. In the next chapter recent evidence on kinship ties is followed by a discussion of isolation and loneliness in modern society and the implications of privacy concerns for informal care. The aim is not to provide a fully rounded account of existing patterns of informal care, which is anyway available elsewhere for kin (Willmott, 1986a; Allan, 1985), neighbours (Bulmer, 1986a) and friends

(Allan, 1979; Willmott, 1986a). Rather, the aim is to highlight certain specific sociological issues which have a direct bearing on the caring capacity of the community as policy-makers conceive – and misconceive it. Indirectly, the aim serves the purpose of highlighting and beginning to subject to scrutiny the sociological assumptions with which policy-makers operate.

THE PRIMARY GROUP

'Community care' appeals to the idea of a past society with a dense interlocking network of personal ties in which people took responsibility for each other and social support was available for those in a state of dependency. Despite the undoubted strengths of 'community studies' (cf. Bell and Newby, 1971), 'community' has proved to be an unsatisfactory concept for getting a grasp upon these local tightly-knit informal social ties. This is mainly as a result of sociological approaches which erected the rural and the urban as polar types and tied social relationships directly to particular geographical relationships. If one conceptualizes social relationships in terms of the 'primary group' instead of 'community', many of these difficulties are greatly diminished. A return to the sociology of the primary group, neglected for some years by sociologists, is in order and likely to yield benefits. More attention needs to be given to the familiar distinctions between primary group relationships and institutionalized relationships, between personal relationships and socially structured relationships.

Traditional locality studies show that people interact with one another in a variety of different settings, at work, in commerce, through religious or political organizations, or other voluntary associations, as well as through informal ties among friends, neighbours and kin. Many such social ties, like those of the workplace or the voluntary association, are structured and institutionalized. There are roles, offices, formal rules and patterns of expectations which govern how people act in those settings. The personal or primordial ties or primary group members, on the other hand, are established on the basis of affect, tradition or propinquity (in the case of neighbours). Primary groups are also a way of understanding informal processes which operate within formal settings.

The sociological study of the primary group may be justified in terms of its salience for people's lives (cf. Cooley, 1909, pp. 23–31). We need to take more account than we do of the ordinary person's attachment 'to his mates, to his pub, to his family, to his petty vanities in his job, to his vulgar gratifications, to his concern for the improvement of his conditions of life' (Shils, 1957, p. 131). Primordial and personal affinities are of demonstrable importance even in formal contexts such as workplaces.[1] If the rural–urban continuum is in disgrace, there is still much interest in contemporary sociology in the local versus the national or, in a different way, micro-sociology versus macro-sociology (Knorr-Cetina and Cicourel, 1981).

The personal ties of geographical propinquity between neighbours are one example of primary group relationships. Despite a decline in people's local attachments, they remain significant in certain types of locality and in all localities potentially of importance at times of social stress. Their study was a traditional theme of British community studies. 'Economics is all about how people make choices. Sociology is all about why they don't have choices to make.' Duesenberry's aphorism (1960, p. 233) hits the nail on the head so far as the study of neighbouring is concerned, for one's neighbours are, by definition, those over whom one has no degree of choice or control. They are given by the facts of physical propinquity. It does not follow, of course, that one necessarily has social contact with them.[2]

A major benefit of shifting the emphasis from the study of 'community' to the study of the primary group – whether made up of neighbours, friends or kin – is that it gets away from the metaphysical problem of community. The study of neighbours, for example, indeed focuses upon the social relationships of geographical propinquity and certainly the term 'neighbour' needs careful definition – there are degrees of nearness and farness (cf. Bulmer, 1986a, pp. 18–22) – but it does not involve the reification of a geographical or structural entity which has proved so problematical in the case of 'community'. To be sure, the existence of ties between neighbours remains empirically problematical, and it may well be the case that, in certain settings, for certain sectors of the population, ties between neighbours are slight or relatively unimportant. Ways of life, indeed, do not coincide with settlement patterns, however, in studying neighbours one is not studying settlement patterns but social networks and the ways in which people construct their primary group relationships. 'Social network', indeed, is a term that has come to be used extensively in studies of social care. It will be discussed further in Chapter 4.

The study of personal ties between neighbours also meshes easily with the study of kin relations and friendship. Phenomena of 'neighbouring', the actual patterns of social interaction observed among neighbours, are potentially important for the provision of social care. Such social behaviour can be more fruitfully understood by looking at relations between neighbours alongside ties between kin and ties of friendship, as types of primary group relationship, than it can be trying to integrate the study of neighbours into traditional urban sociology (cf. Willmott, 1986a). These comments relate to neighbours and neighbouring. The concept of 'neighbourhood' is much more problematical, and open to many of the same objections that have been directed against the concept of 'community' (cf. Dennis, 1958).

A range of variables – social class, sex, age, ethnicity, stage of life cycle, mobility experience, type of neighbourhood – influence the actual patterns of neighbourly contact and involvement, but there is no evidence that neighbouring has ceased to be a significant social relationship (cf. Keller, 1968; Bulmer, 1986a). An approach formulated in terms of primary group relationships seems more fruitful than one tied, problematically, to geographical space. 'Community', because of the legacy from Toennies, carries the implication that phenomena subsumed under it are local. 'Primary group' carries no such implication, and research shows that kinship and friendship ties extend over long distances. Such personal ties can then be compared with ties of neighbouring, as a fruitful way of judging the nature, strength and intensity of each.

A shift of emphasis to the primary group also permits one to take account of other types of primordial tie such as ethnic or racial attachment. Relationships among and between members of different racial and ethnic minority groups at the local level are not institutionalized and are frequently face-to-face, but they are not necessarily tied to the local level.

There are various conditions which facilitate the growth of primary groups. Bates and Babchuk (1961) suggested that the key features of belonging to a primary group are that membership is to be enjoyed for its own sake, and that a strong affective element is present in the ties between members. Structural factors are secondary, groups being more likely to become primary the smaller they are, the longer established they are, the more frequently members interact and the more homogeneous they are. It is the character of the relationship which is the central component in the definition. The structural factors are all facilitating conditions, the presence of any one of which does not by itself create a primary group.

It is this insight which has been lost sight of in much of the literature of urban sociology and the study of the spatial distribution of social phenomena. In some of its manifestations, such as the political economy of regionalism, either informal ties were ignored altogether or treated merely as the product of larger social forces. Theories which emphasize spatial or structural determinism inevitably play down these defining characteristics of primary groups, treating them instead as products of settings which create small-scale, face-to-face, intense social interaction. Instead, it may be more fruitful to ask in what situations in modern industrial society are personal relationships based on a primary group pursued for their own sake on an affective basis; how large do they loom in people's lives; and what implications do they have for other spheres of social behaviour – such as social care?

GEMEINSCHAFT AND GESELLSCHAFT

To assess the part played by personal relationships, some sense of the direction of social change is needed. What tools are available to understand societal change? The best known sociological concepts referring to different types of society are the German terms *gemeinschaft* and *gesellschaft*, originally formulated by Ferdinand Toennies and translated, not altogether accurately, as 'community' and 'association'. Toennies sought to distinguish between social relationships which are small-scale, personal, and particular from those which were large-scale, impersonal and more universal. The former were more likely to be found at earlier stages of social development, while the latter were increasingly characteristic of an industrialized and urbanized society. These features are familiar, as are the usual problems, such as whether the distinction was intended as a typology or an hypothesis about the course of historical development.

The importance of the distinction in relation to informal social care is that *gemeinschaft* was based upon affective and traditional ties, and *gesellschaft* upon individualism, contractualism and the rational pursuit of interest. Toennies suggested that European society had developed from (1) unions of *gemeinschaft* to (2) associations of *gemeinschaft*, then to (3) associations of *gesellschaft* and finally to (4) unions of *gesellschaft*. This four fold typology has considerable relevance to informal care. What did he mean by each term? The first type corresponded to what we mean by personal ties.

> The prototype of all unions of *gemeinschaft* is the family. By birth man enters these relationships: free rational will can determine his remaining within the family, but the very existence of the relationship itself is not dependent on his full rational will. The three pillars of *gemeinschaft* – blood, place (land) and mind, or kinship, neighbourhood and friendship – are all encompassed in the family, but the first of them is the constituting element of it. (Toennies, 1957, p. 192)

His second type, associations of *gemeinschaft*, are based on common work or calling, and thus on common beliefs with a traditional or affective component. They extend beyond purely personal ties to bodies such as guilds, fellowships, churches and holy orders. Many attempts to formalize informal social care, as in neighbourhood care schemes, are attempts – very often unsuccessfully – to create associations of *gemeinschaft*.

His third type, associations of *gesellschaft*, represent the epitomy of rationality and calculation, with activity restricted to definite means in pursuit of a definite end. Their embodiment is the large corporation or public bureaucracy, run according to formal rules. Action does not occur on the basis of personal ties. 'Here everybody is by himself and isolated, and there exists a condition of tension against all others' (Toennies, 1957, p. 65).

Toennies, however, suggested a fourth type: unions of

gesellschaft. Whereas the first three types point to growing individualization, impersonality and competition, the fourth type represents an attempt to reintroduce into the public or private bureaucracy some of the personal ties characteristic of *gemeinschaft*, through human relations, or social insurance. The responsibilities of government for social care may also be interpreted in this light. A personal relationship of caring is involved, even though the framework within which it is provided is a formal and impersonal one. The ties developed between district nurses or home helps and their clients are indicative of such a modification.

Treated as a simple dichotomy, *gemeinschaft* and *gesellschaft* are of limited conceptual use. The finer distinctions between associations of *gemeinschaft* and unions of *gesellschaft*, however, are of considerable value when thinking about the types of social care available, for they differentiate between the bases on which care may be provided, for example, between voluntary care of a formally organized kind, paid statutory care by local people, and commercially provided care.

Associated with the transition from *gemeinschaft* to *gesellschaft* is the postulation of the breakdown of the primary group and the rise of mass society in its impersonal, rationalized urban form. The primary group may be defined as 'a group characterized by a high degree of solidarity, informality in the code of rules which regulate the behavior of its members, and autonomy in the creation of these rules' (Shils, 1951, p. 44). This solidarity involves a close identification of the members with one another, and with any symbols of the group which have developed. Some groups are characterized by small size and face-to-face relations, but this is not necessarily a feature. The most important primary groups, according to Charles H. Cooley who developed the term, are 'the family, the play-group of children, and the neighbourhood or community group of elders. These are practically universal, belonging to all times and all stages of development; and are accordingly a chief basis of what is universal in human nature and human ideals' (Cooley, 1909, p. 24).

For social care, those sociological theories which discern a historical trend toward the disintegration of primary groups in the rural and village *gemeinschaft* and the rise of impersonal *gesellschaft* in modern urban society are of particular interest. There are a variety of such theories. Sir Henry Maine's transition from status to contract, Emile Durkheim's from mechanical to organic solidarity and Max Weber's from traditional to rational-legal authority, postulated a necessary historical transition from the simple to the complex, homogeneous to heterogeneous, undifferentiated to differentiated. Such theories are significant for the consideration of community care because ideas about long-term social development underlie the discussion. There are frequently implicit comparisons or generalizations, for example, looking back to a 'golden age' or postulating 'the decline of community' as a long-term trend. Nineteenth-century theorists not only described the transition from a small-scale face-to-face society to a rationalized, more impersonal one, but suggested, implicitly or explicitly, an evolutionary historical development toward complex, large-scale, differentiated societies based on rational calculation. Such a transition was associated with changes in urban form, as the individual moved from the village *gemeinschaft* to the impersonal and abstract world of the city.

Georg Simmel caught the phenomenon well in his essay on 'The Metropolis and Mental Life'. He contrasted the small intellectual horizons, the constraints and the unspecialized character of the village or small town with the broader intellectual horizons, freedom, specialized and impersonal character of the city. One form which this takes in the city is a blasé mental attitude, another is reserve as a form of self-preservation adopted by the city dweller. 'As a result of this reserve, we frequently do not even know by sight those who have been our neighbours for years. It is this reserve which in the eyes of small-town people makes us appear to be cold and heartless' (Simmel, 1950, p. 415). These ideas were also explored by Robert Park at the University of Chicago, and by Louis Wirth in his influential article on 'Urbanism as a way of life' (1938) which developed a polar contrast between the small scale and the large scale, rural and urban social relationships.

In a slightly different form the contrast was also incorporated into theories of mass society. Such theories emphasized the impersonality of modern urban life, its anarchic individualism, the consequent isolation and alienation, and the peculiar mental qualities enhanced by a concern with money and abstraction. This disorganization created by industrialization was contrasted with the social features of traditional society, which stressed the

importance of the primary group – the family, small occupation..
groups and guilds of the church – all characterized by face-to-face
relationships and strong mutual identification enhanced by their
small size and physical proximity. Behind such theories –
whether of the left or the right – lay 'a romantic notion of the past
that sees society as having once been made up of small "organic"
communities that were shattered by industrialism and modern
life, and replaced by an 'atomistic' society which is unable to
provide the basic gratifications and call forth the loyalties that the
older communities knew' (Bell, 1956, p. 77).

SOCIAL CHANGE

General and relatively abstract though it is, the theme of social
change in the types of social tie characteristic of industrial societies
needs some consideration, for it looms large in discussion of the
scope for informal social care, past and present. The 'decline of
community' thesis was indeed built into Louis Wirth's influential
article on the city. Under urban conditions, he suggested, social
relations were 'impersonal, superficial, transitory and segmen-
tal'. Functional roles were highly specialized and interdependent.
'The distinctive features of the urban mode of life are the substitution of secondary for primary contacts, the weakening of bonds
of kinship, and the declining social significance of the family, the
disappearance of the neighbourhood, and the undermining of the
traditional basis of social solidarity' (Wirth, 1938). With this
collapse of *gemeinschaft*, Wirth suggested that 'competition and
formal control mechanisms [would have to] furnish the substitute
for the bonds of solidarity that are relied upon to hold a folk
society together'. The echoes of Simmel were not accidental, for
Wirth's mentor, Robert Park, had been influenced by Simmel
during his time in Germany, and Simmel had had some early
influence upon American sociology (Levine *et al.*, 1976).

The theme of the 'decline of community' has been pervasive in
twentieth-century sociology. Charles Cooley, in formulating his
ideas about the primary group, discerned such a trend:

In our own life, the intimacy of the neighbourhood has been
broken up by the growth of an intricate mesh of wider contacts

...us strangers to people who live in the same house.
...the country, the same principle is at work, dimin-
...economic and spiritual community with our neigh-
...Cooley, 1909, p. 26)

...of the transition from *gemeinschaft* to *gesellschaft* were
...on the belief that 'community' was breaking down. As
Toennies put it, in *gemeinschaft* people 'remain essentially united
in spite of all separating factors, whereas in *gesellschaft* they are
essentially separated in spite of all uniting factors' (Toennies,
1957, p. 65).

The theme has also been present in the writing of American
history. Thomas Bender has analyzed how a number of noted
studies share

> what I will call a narrative form that is remarkably similar to
> what one finds in Wirthian formulations of social theory. The
> narrative is shaped by unrelenting community decline . . .
> what is casually assumed in them to be a proper narrative
> structure is based upon an unexamined sociological idea. . . .
> Collectively [these studies] portray the collapse of community
> during the lives of several successive generations of Americans.
> One is impelled to ask: Which study accurately captures the
> moment of collapse? How many times can community collapse
> in America? (Bender, 1978, pp. 45–6).[3]

This is illuminating in itself of the pitfalls of totalistic theories
which postulate transition from one type of society to another
completely different society. Not only is this logically unsatisfactory – elements of *gemeinschaft* and *gesellschaft* may (and indeed do)
coexist in the same society at one point in time – but, as noted
earlier, the considerable empirical evidence of the persistence of
gemeinschaft within urban *gesellschaft* has undermined the typology. Bender's study also makes the point, which is applicable to
the field of 'community care', that 'the sociological formulation
(of the decline of community) seems to have been absorbed into
the working assumptions of historians. At a fairly deep level of
consciousness, it has often provided an *a priori* interpretive framework for their scholarship' (Bender, 1978, p. 46). The process of
'cultural seepage' that brought sociological theory to influence

major American historical writing has parallels in other fields, including social welfare policy.

On the one hand, community care policies are strongly imbued with the idea of the decline of community, while on the other they embody a considerable element of nostalgia for that lost world and the belief that it is possible to regain those sorts of communal social relationships. The theme of community lost and regained will be taken up again in Chapter 4.

Theories of overall historical development provide a framework within which to interpret social change. There is no substitute, however, for an account informed both by ideas *and* empirical evidence, and it is this which has been lacking as 'community care' policies have been gaining in popularity. Assumptions about the trends of historical development are powerful underlying features in notions of community care. So what can one say, briefly and in a compressed summary, about these trends? At what periods, for example, was the self-sufficient and all-embracing traditional village community typical? Although one may have to go back to feudal society to find it, one found there individual settlements to a large extent isolated from the rest of the world.

> Men . . . shrank from those repeated comings and goings within a narrow radius which in other civilisations form the texture of daily life; and this was especially the case of humble folk of settled occupation. The result was an ordering of the scheme of human relationships quite different from anything we know today. . . . Between two inhabited centres quite close to each other the connections were much rarer, the isolation of their inhabitants infinitely greater than would be the case in our own day. If, according to the angle from which it is viewed, the civilization of feudal Europe appears sometimes remarkably universalist, sometimes particularist in the extreme, the principal source of this contradiction lay in the conditions of communication: conditions which favoured the distant propagation of very general currents of influence as much as they discouraged, in any particular place, the standardizing effects of neighbourly intercourse. (Bloch, 1962, p. 64)

In such a society, assistance in times of adversity came from one's kin in the locality and other local residents. As Charles Cooley observed:

> of the neighbourhood group it may be said, in general, that from the time men formed permanent settlements upon the land, down, at least, to the rise of modern industrial cities, it has played a main part in the primary, heart to heart life of the people. Among our teutonic forefathers *the village community was apparently the chief sphere of sympathy and mutual aid for the commons* all through the 'dark' and middle ages, and for many purposes it remains so in rural districts at the present day (italics added). (1909, p. 25)

This ideal picture (not an ideal type) has held powerful sway, just as the rural idea holds powerful sway in British urban sociology (Glass, 1955) and in social thought in Britain more generally (Williams, 1973). The village has been seen as the epitomy of the caring, concerned community in feudal times, within the constraints of lord and vassal relationship. Vassalage, indeed, was a system that formally recognized the personal tie between lord and vassal and acknowledged, moreover, unlike slavery and serfdom, that it was a reciprocal relationship, albeit between people of different social status. Though its prime objective was to ensure military service, it also implied responsibility for caring for the injured, ill and aged. Indeed, 'the relationships of personal dependence . . . made their entry into history as a sort of substitute for, or complement to, the solidarity of the family, which had ceased to be fully effective. . . . In relation to the lord, the vassal remained a sort of supplementary relative, his duties as well as his rights being the same as those of relatives by blood' (Bloch, 1962, p. 224). For the lower social orders, it was a relationship within a restricted geographical locality, the estate of the lord.

From the early modern period onwards, feudalism gave way to more varied forms of landownership with free tenants, peasant farmers or agricultural labourers, to a large extent confined to the locality and more or less under the sway of the local landowner. The ideal was that of the beneficent paternalism of the landowner towards his villagers, though the reality was often much less than this. Nevertheless, the idea of local self-sufficiency and mutual aid remained a strong one. English Poor Relief, indeed, was a system built upon the assumption that a person's place of birth was the place responsible for looking after that person in times of need, destitution or indigence.

With the coming of industrialism, rural dwellers migrated to the towns and lived there in conditions of poverty, overcrowding and relative impersonality that was a world removed from the rural village. Yet in these unpropitious circumstances there developed quite strong informal ties through which self-help and mutual aid were provided. Some such ties were developed through formal institutions such as Friendly Societies; the majority, however, were provided on the basis of personal ties between kin and neighbours. Indeed, the existence of such ties in strength is one of the reasons for doubting the Wirthian theory of modern urbanism, since it so severely modifies ideas of the impersonality, superficiality and transitory nature of urban contacts.

Consider the following description of neighbourhood care in London in the early years of the twentieth century. Here is little support for Simmel's picture of the city as cultivating a blasé and detached individualism, in which people bumped together like molecules. Powerful links between both men and their work-mates, and between women and their kin and neighbours – links often involving substantial exchanges of services and money – bound together households in the same local area.

> Poor women did indeed share extensively and unsentimentally. Small sums of money, like a penny for the gas, were passed back and forth between households, and even on these cash-poor streets, women could launch collections toward such major expenses as funerals. Domestic paraphernalia circulated too between women: linen, washtubs, clothing or other pawnable items which the borrower could use to raise immediate cash. In emergencies like serious illness or eviction, neighbours could be counted on for major services, something not contingent on having maintained cordial ties, but on the obligations people viewed as part of 'the neighbourhood role'. Women giving birth, and their children, would be cared for. Battered wives could get shelter for a night. . . . Custom reserved special treatment for the sick. Neighbourhood women did their laundry, built (and provided) their fires, prepared their meals. (Ross, 1983, p. 6)

Such self-help networks at the local level were a realistic response to low incomes, economic adversity and unpredictable domestic crisis. In the absence of state support for relief in the home of illness, old age or unemployment, the 'safety net' for most families was the neighbourhood 'A family who have lived for years in one street are recognised up and down the length of that street as people to be helped in times of trouble' (Pember-Reeves, 1913, p. 39). There were limits to the extent of aid. Neighbours were helpful in meeting small-scale or very short-term material needs, and to deal with various forms of domestic crisis for a week or two. Neighbours, however, could not provide adequate support for a household with too few wage earners – unmarried or deserted women with small children. Widows and the elderly were more likely to have to move to the workhouse. Other forms of care were commonly provided on a neighbourhood basis. Neighbours and even neighbourhoods could act as auxiliary parents, keeping an eye on children when their parents were not there. When a mother of young children was ill, neighbours as well as extended kin would help out.

In the twentieth century, this pattern continued with recognizable general features. The traditional working class neighbourhood has been documented in literature and in the famous sociological community studies of Bethnal Green, North Wales, St. Ebbe's in the old centre of Oxford, 'Ashton', a Yorkshire mining village, Dagenham and elsewhere. David Lockwood's characterization of traditional single-industry communities based on coal, steel or shipbuilding, catches the main elements of such neighbourhoods.

> The existence of such closely-knit cliques of friends, workmates, neighbours and relatives is the hall-mark of the traditional working-class community. The values expressed through these social networks emphasise mutual aid in everyday life and the obligation to join in a gregarious pattern of leisure. . . . As a form of social life, this communal sociability has a ritualistic quality, creating a high moral density and reinforcing sentiments of belongingness to a work-dominated collectivity (Lockwood, 1966, p. 251).

Localitites were permeated with dense, complex and extensive social networks that evoked sufficient commitment from residents to meet a high proportion of local needs for care.

The appeal to 'community' implicit in community care policies is an amalgam of elements from the image of the traditional village on the one hand and the historical features of these urban working-class neighbourhoods on the other. Not only do they sit rather uneasily together, but their social basis is frequently idealized and romanticized. At a popular level this occurs in stereotypes of the idyllic rural society, but it can be perpetuated also in sociological accounts of the solid, tightly-knit urban working class 'community'. As Philip Abrams suggested,

> The problem with the traditional neighbourhood type of social network is not that it is a thing of the past, rapidly being eliminated by the forces of social change, but that when one considers the social conditions that made it possible one is forced to the conclusion that on balance it is probably rather undesirable. This is a matter of looking at the social *contexts* of the networks rather than at the caring and supportive relationships within them. Internally, the networks of the traditional neighbourhood were indeed marked by collective attachment, reciprocity and trust. Externally, they were no less plainly marked by constraint, isolation and insecurity. Moreover, the internal characteristics were in large measure a product of the external characteristics, a way of life worked out to permit survival in the face of them. The so-called natural helping networks of the traditional neighbourhood – not actually natural at all of course – developed as a response to certain highly specified social conditions which one would not wish to see reproduced today. . . . Reciprocal care between neighbours grows where information and trust are high and where resources for satisfying needs in other ways are low; in relatively isolated, relatively closed and relatively threatened social milieux with highly homogeneous populations (Bulmer, 1986a, pp. 92–3).

It is clear, in the last quarter of the twentieth century, that the tightly-knit networks of early nineteenth-century Preston (Anderson, 1971), early twentieth-century Salford (Roberts, 1971), inter-war Islington (White, 1986) or mid-twentieth century Bethnal Green (Young and Willmott, 1957) are not reliable guides to the character of informal local social relationships at the present day. A recent review of kin relationships (Willmott,

1986a), for example, estimates that only one in eight of the population has members of their extended family living in close geographical propinquity to them.

Philip Abrams contrasted the traditional pattern of neighbourhood relations, as one type of informal care, with what he called 'modern neighbourhoodism'.

> Most neighbourhoods today do not constrain their inhabitants into strongly bonded relationships with one another. Those that do are either exceptional or regrettable. Generally the old equation of problems, resources and closure which produced the diffuse trust and reciprocity of the traditional neighbourhood type networks, within which care in 'critical life situations' could effectively be provided for and by local residents, has plainly collapsed in the face of new social patterns. Most neighbours are not constrained and do not choose to make their friends among their neighbours. Those who do tend to be seeking highly specific solutions to highly specific problems which they cannot solve elsewhere and which make them 'expensive' people to befriend from the point of view of their neighbours (Bulmer, 1986a, p. 94).

CHANGING LOCAL ATTACHMENTS

Changes which have taken place in people's local attachments have considerable implications both for the character of local social networks and for the provision of informal care. Some local kinship ties and gossip persist, but are overlaid by the loosening of the personal ties which in the past bound and constrained most working-class people to their immediate locality. Improved personal transport, notably by motor car or motor bike, is one of the key changes. Car ownership in Britain has risen from 30 per cent in 1961 to 61 per cent in 1984 (Willmott, 1986a, p. 20). People are more mobile. The rapid spread of telephone ownership enables certain activities, particularly contact with kin, to be maintained over considerable distances. Whereas in 1969 only just over one-third of British households had a telephone, the proportion had risen to nearly four-fifths in 1984 (Willmott, 1986a, p. 21).

The loosening of local ties takes several forms. Car ownership in particular has permitted longer journeys to work, although the historical decline of certain industries such as coal, steel, ship-building and textiles, whose workers tended to live in 'occupa-tional communities' near their place of work (cf. Bulmer, 1975), is also part of the explanation of weakening attachment to the locality. Manufacturing and service industries have recruited workers without regard to residence, and increases in distances travelled to work have been gradually taking place over several decades. As in work, so in leisure. The motor car permits a wider range of shopping and recreational activities of a more far flung kind. No longer is the local shop or local club or pub or local cinema or bingo hall the only option available. The growth of large city-centre shopping areas and, more recently, out-of-town centres, some with hypermarkets and all with good parking facilities, has broadened the range of choice in shopping. The motor car permits alternative leisure patterns of a more individu-alized kind, and although collective pursuits continue – the outing of the Darby and Joan club, the visit to the theatre by members of the Townswomen's Guild, the football supporters club going to an away match, or the Sunday angling contest – better transport widens the range of choice available.

People's geographical horizons have widened, too. This is most evident in where people take holidays. Traditional northern coastal resorts such as Skegness, Scarborough, Redcar, Whitley Bay, Largs and Blackpool catered for particular geographical catchment areas of the urban working class. The same was true of Southend, Margate, Brighton, Bognor, Weston-super-Mare and other southern resorts. Many people still holiday there, but the large growth of coach and air travel to resorts in southern Europe, particularly Spain and Greece, has altered both the holiday indus-try and people's experience of other places. Even if British eating and drinking places have been exported to parts of the Spanish coast, the locals do speak a different language. Another major factor in broadening people's horizons has been the spread of the mass media, in particular television. While the popular press now takes a more international interest in the news, it is television which has expanded people's perceptions of regions and strata of British society other than their own, as well as of the world overseas.

It would be possible to avail oneself of all these opportunities to learn more of the wider world, and yet remain rooted in a particular place, perhaps where one was born. There is a well-established correlation between education and geographical mobility. The further one progresses through the education system, the more likely one is to move away from the area where one was brought up. To the extent that the occupational structure has been changing, and non-manual positions increasing at the expense of manual jobs, there will be rather greater intergenerational movement between strata, and a consequent greater geographical mobility among the upwardly mobile children of the working class. Once established in non-manual work, expectations of geographical mobility are higher, either voluntarily or as a condition of employment, in occupations such as banking, the sales side of commerce, industries with multiple plants and teaching and hospital medicine.

Following Young and Willmott's 'Principle of stratified diffusion' (Young and Willmott, 1975, pp. 19–22), the traditionally higher geographical mobility among the middle classes is now being followed by greater degrees of mobility among the working class. Long distance mobility – whether inter-war movement from north to south to growth centres such as Welwyn, Slough or Coventry, or after the war to new industrial centres such as Luton or Stevenage, or between coalfields as a result of pit closures, or short-term movement to the oil rigs or the continent of Europe in search of higher paid work – has always been unusual. What has occurred on a considerable scale, however, partly due to urban renewal but also to a greater willingness to move some distance from the areas of origin and kin, has been short-distance mobility to new housing on the periphery of large conurbations, to new towns, or to middle-class suburbs.

A tightly-knit city has been gradually converted into a looser region. Compression has given way to expansion. More people have been able both to remain within the job and collective life of the city and to gain a .urchase on the new provinces because their frontiers have been steadily rolled back. . . . In London, richer people have, in accord with the Principle, led the way, and others, too, have gained an advantage from the extra space that transport has brought within their reach. (Young and Willmott, 1975, pp. 49–50)

A major consequence of this pattern of urban change has been a transformation from working-class kinship ties which are locally based and tightly knit to a pattern where people's kin ties are more dispersed and loosely knit. A recent estimate suggests that about half the population now have kinship links with the extended family of this type (Willmott, 1986a, p. 27). What was previously a characteristic middle-class pattern (cf. C. Bell, 1968) has now become characteristic also of sections of the working class. Contact with kin – particularly between parents and grown-up children themselves married, is maintained by the motor car and telephone. In times of need, one can travel to the other, but day-to-day local contact has more typically been replaced by week-to-week contact from a distance.

Such shifts in urban social structure have increased the range of choices available to many working class families. To be sure, the constraints of the labour market and labour power which they command is a basic restraint upon the income which can be earned. How that income is spent, however, is a matter for much greater choice than in the past, and many activities are pursued outside the locality because of greater mobility. Suzanne Keller's generalization has stood the test of time well: 'Local self-sufficiency and local self-reliance are diminishing everywhere. Concentration on the local area seems to be most strongly correlated with lack of alternatives' (Keller, 1968, p. 116).

One must remember, however, that the above generalizations do not apply uniformly to all sections of society. The locality remains the centre of their social world for most young children, for their mothers, and for many elderly people, particularly among the over 75s who are unsteady or infirm. The poorer sections of society – the unemployed, chronically sick, single parents, and those in low paid manual work – lack the financial resources to benefit from the range of choices available, in particular because they do not have cars or spare money for public transport fares. Their lives are likely to be more circumscribed and more confined to the immediate locality. As Young and Willmott observed, 'to the poor, the region meant nothing' (Young and Willmott, 1975, p. 61).

Some sections of the population, therefore, still live, and maintain a majority of their significant social ties, within a narrow locality. In contrast to the traditional neighbourhood, however, many others in the locality are not oriented to the locality in the same way, so that the traditional solidarity and mutual aid of the past cannot be drawn upon to the same extent. If one considers, for example, the nuclear family with young children, mother and children will tend to centre their lives upon the locality and be involved in ties of reciprocal aid with neighbours. But demographic change toward smaller families means that such families are now in a minority in the society.

> Small families with closely-spaced births, coupled with greatly extended life-spans, means child-bearing and -rearing have become truncated, sharply contracted as a phase of life that previously supported a significant proportion of adulthood. Only one in four American households now include even one dependent age child. At a societal level, this may carry with it an erosion of a major source of social integration. (Rossi, 1984, p. 4)

Because of such demographic changes, as well as social and economic change, personal ties between co-residents are much weaker than they used to be, for many local people's most significant personal ties lie elsewhere. Hence, appeals by policy-makers to 'the community' as a basis for care lack reality to the extent that the locality is not a tightly-knit, highly integrated social network.

The idea of network will be discussed further in Chapter 4, but one way of characterizing the transition described here is the shift from multiplex to single-stranded relationships. In a long-established neighbourhood with a high degree of interaction, people belong to multiple, overlapping networks, based on kinship, being neighbours, long residence, common schooling, common involvement in leisure pursuits, perhaps common religious affiliations, political or voluntary association membership, and even – in the case of occupational communities – work. People have ties with other people not just in one sphere but in several; thus their relationships are multiplex. With greater mobility and choice, such multiplex relationships weaken and disappear. In the image of urban man put forward by Wirth and Simmel, he was rootless and detached and interacted with different people in different settings: at work, in the family, in leisure pursuits, with neighbours, and so on. Such relationships are single-stranded, with no overlap between different spheres. The tightly-knit network and the atomized individual are ideal-typical extremes, but there has been movement along the continuum between them from a more multiplex to a more single-stranded pattern of relationships. If, as has been argued, multiplex local networks are more sustaining of informal care, then a move, however incomplete, toward single-strandedness in personal ties suggests an attenuation of resources available for informal care.

PRIVATIZATION

As important as changes within the locality are changes in the nature of the family itself and the social relationships and outlook upon the world of family members. For, while the activities of the neighbourhood are generally public, those of the family are private. With marriage, a house

> becomes again the centre of people's lives. Space, privacy and storage room – indoors and outdoors – baths, hot water, properly equipped kitchens and a parking space, become urgent necessities. The neighbourhood and the accessibility of its [facilities] takes on a new importance. If the roof leaks you can no longer escape by moving; if the woman next door bangs angrily on the wall, you can no longer simply bang back. You have to live with it – or your wife does – all day. The security and privacy of this home and the right to go on living peacefully in it are the foundations of the family's happiness (Donnison, 1967, p. 277).

The relationship between this private realm and the public sphere of work, neighbourhood and recreation outside the home is an important one for informal social care, both in terms of the informal relationships which people build up with others which potentially may form a basis for mutual aid, and in determining who is admitted to the home (the private realm) on the basis of intimacy. The phenomenon of privatization has been examined most thoroughly in the sociological literature in relation to affluent manual workers, who exhibited an instrumental work orientation, and adopted a pattern of life centred on, and largely restricted to, the home and the conjugal family, restricting the scope of communal sociability outside the family. This links with the thesis of the 'decline of community', but in the form of a more specific hypothesis that for some sections of the population their range of informal social contacts is becoming more restricted. Thus it is argued that 'recent changes both in the nature of local communities and in patterns of consumption are combining to produce increasingly privatised life-styles and increasingly individualised home- or family-centred social identities based on them' (Newby *et al.*, 1985, p. 95).

Contemporary commentators on social ills clearly consider that trends toward privatization affect the quality of life in British cities. The Archbishop of Canterbury's Commission on the city (1985), for example, observed that

> a significant number of people in the inner city and outer estates are friendless and desperately lonely . . . large numbers of people in urban priority areas are deprived of 'community' by being excluded by poverty or unemployment from fulfilling relationships in their neighbourhood. . . . Poor people can be forced into isolated and lonely lives . . . where sound networks have not developed to meet human needs for interaction. . . . The concern was rather with a 'privatization' which is inflicted upon people by circumstances. . . . The result is an acute form of urban deprivation: deprivation of relatedness, of esteem (quoted in Thomas, 1986, p. 95).

'Privatization' is thus a matter of policy significance as well as a purely sociological issue.

Like *gemeinschaft* this process of privatization may be considered over a long time-scale. Philip Aries has suggested a long-term trend of the insulation of the family at the expense of sociability.

> Starting in the eighteenth century, people began defending themselves against a society whose constant intercourse had hitherto been the source of education, reputation and wealth. . . . Everywhere it reinforced private life at the expense of neighbourly relationships, friendships and traditional contacts (Aries, 1962, pp. 393–4).

In his study of Chicago in the 1860s and 1870s, Richard Sennett argued that 'the home had, in some way, become the focus for a new kind of intense family life, a life that was private and isolated'

(Sennett, 1970, p. 50). M. J. Daunton discerns a similar process at work among some sections of the British working class around the same period.

> On the most general level, there was a re-orientation of working-class culture from being work-centred to home-centred. Of course this was not a uniform trend; it applied less to mining towns, for example, than to large industrial towns where work-place and residence were distant. But generally, shorter working hours and increased real wages eroded work-centred culture and increased the role of the home as the centre of life. (Daunton, 1983, p. 224)

Improved real wages in the last quarter of the nineteenth century meant that workers could afford better accommodation and higher consumption standards within the home.

In the nineteenth century, two urban trends facilitated this social change. The layout of Victorian cities began to change, from a closed to a more open layout of continuous streets; at the same time each dwelling was encapsulated more sharply by the boundary between private and public space being clearly defined (for example, by communal facilities being abandoned, giving each dwelling its own back yard and privy, and so on). Secondly, the internal facilities of houses were gradually improved by the progressive installation of gas and sanitation, making dwellings more habitable. 'Daily life became less public and less communal, more private and more introverted' (Daunton, 1983, p. 232). Interestingly, these trends were associated with the growth of working-class political rights and citizenship, and the cultural, political and economic integration of the working class into the nation-state, both through trade unionism, self-help organizations and the extension of the franchise.

Nevertheless, despite these trends toward home-based activities, localities remained close-knit both because their inhabitants were geographically confined to them and those who lived there did take part in public activities on a regular basis, whether in the pub, club, chapel, music hall, cinema, football ground, corner shop or just on the street. It is only in the second half of the twentieth century that 'privatization' has come to have the particular connotations of withdrawal from the public sphere and attenuation of community ties. It is important to be clear that there may be a decline in the salience of the locality without privatization resulting. It may be simply that people's social ties are more widely dispersed geographically. People's social networks may include some who live locally and others who live at varying distances away from that locality. The neighbourhood is thus no longer a cohesive unit, but individuals need not be privatized as a result. They may simply have a more widely spread range of contacts (Allan, 1985, p. 76).

Privatization also has two dimensions which should be distinguished, depending on whether one is looking outward or inward from the family. Outwardly, the concept postulates a weakening of local informal social ties, with both kin and non kin, resulting in isolation for the individual household. Inwardly, it draws attention to changes in the character of family life, the greater salience of the domestic sphere for men as well as women, and the decreasing significance of relationships with those outside the family. Change along one of these dimensions does not necessarily entail change in the other. There is a difference, for example, between home-centredness more characteristic of affluent manual workers (e.g. Goldthorpe *et al.*, 1969) and family-centredness characteristic of sections of the mobile middle class (e.g. C. Bell, 1968). In both cases, the inward dimension of privatization was evident. In the working class case, however, privatization took the form of cutting off many external ties, whereas in the mobile middle class there developed a loose-knit local network of informal ties through associational activities, while close links (hence family-centredness) were maintained with geographically distant kin. In the former case isolation was the result, whereas in the latter there was involvement in a network whose heart lay outside the locality.

There are several different aspects to trends toward privatization which need disentangling. The first concerns the contribution of material changes to an increase in home-centredness. Familiar features of consumption behaviour to some extent explain the changes which have occurred in the relationship between families and other non-kin in their localities. One is the rise of owner-occupation and the decline of privately rented housing. With owner-occupiers now constituting three-fifths of the population, this encourages more attention to be paid to the home and an economic and psychological interest in maintenance of the fabric. The growth of do-it-yourself is one sign of this. The spread of consumer goods has made it possible both to lead a more home-centred life and to improve the quality of that life. Thus, the near universality of television in the home, the high proportions of homes with central heating, refrigerators and washing machines, the sizeable minority with freezers and dishwashers indicates the improved amenity standards which families enjoy. Home-centredness is encouraged by making the home more comfortable and congenial.

Television has also made a great difference to family entertainment. Before its advent, millions went out regularly to the cinema, whereas now a considerable proportion of time is spent viewing at home. The video boom has enhanced the appeal of home entertainment by making home movies available. And such entertainment arguably reinforces home-centredness, since it brings different members of the family together around the screen.

The changes wrought by the motor car and telephone have already been discussed. These are also aspects of privatization. The motor car grants greater mobility, but also insulates the family from wider social contacts in a way that the bus and train, particularly if boarded in one's own locality, do not.

> We seek a private house, a private means of transportation, a private garden, a private laundry, self-service stores and do-it-yourself skills of every kind. An enormous technology seems to have set itself the task of making it unnecessary for one human being to ask anything of another in the course of going about his daily business (Slater, 1970, p. 70)

The telephone also permits social ties to be maintained other than on a face-to-face basis, and for the individual who so chooses to reduce or eliminate social contacts with neighbours and other local residents. Unlike the car, the telephone facilitates privatization but can hardly be said to be a cause of it.

In observing the operation of the principle of stratified diffusion in operation once again, some have argued that what is happening is that home-centred leisure patterns, historically more characteristic of the middle classes, are now diffusing, aided by technological innovation, to the working class. The argument is put most sharply in relation to affluent manual workers. Gold-thorpe and Lockwood's classic study in Luton showed that while the social lives of affluent semi-skilled workers were centred on, and largely restricted to, the home and the conjugal family, this was not so much a sign of incipient 'middle classness' as a response to geographical mobility, separation from kin, an instrumental orientation to well paid work, often on shifts, in modern plants, and an adaptation to the strains and stresses of this new life style. The Luton workers chose to devote time to home and family rather than to wider social contacts, in order to achieve a higher material standard of living. Paradoxically, had they been adopting middle-class norms, they would have been expected to adopt a *less* privatized life style, cultivating social contacts outside the home and joining voluntary associations, neither of which Luton workers tended to do (Goldthorpe *et al.*, 1969, pp. 97–108).

Among the working class, status distinctions have always existed, whether between 'respectable' and 'rough' families or between supervisory and skilled workers on the one hand and the semi-skilled and unskilled on the other. Some families who considered themselves higher in status 'kept themselves to themselves'. This was particularly marked in the case of those in supervisory and junior management positions in single-industry communities. What one may be witnessing is an extension of such a desire 'to preserve the opacity of their domestic lives' (Dennis, 1963) more widely through the working class. It is important, however, to be clear about the basis on which this rests.

The Affluent Worker approach has been criticized for emphasizing excessive geographical mobility at the expense of wider economic changes. Quite high levels of geographical mobility were experienced within communities based on communal solidarity – for example, mining communities (Bulmer, 1977, p. 61 ff.). It is not clear that geographical mobility alone – resulting in attenuation of extended kin ties and more 'companionate' marriage, and leading to instrumental work attitudes – is an adequate explanation of the process of privatization (cf. Newby *et al.*, 1985, p. 98). Nor is the alternative view, postulating the increasingly alienating character of work which causes workers to shift their central life interests to the non-work sphere and redefining achievement in terms of greater personal possessions, a convincing alternative (cf. Chinoy, 1955; Berger, 1960).

What has changed during the last thirty years is the industrial distribution of the working class. The decline of traditional industries has clearly undermined the economic base for the more tightly knit occupational communities, while more recently de-industrialization has reduced the numbers employed in older manufacturing industry. A widening of the geographical area within which the journey to work is undertaken, facilitated by the motor car, is a more significant change than long-distance movement in itself.

Trends toward privatization are also explicable in terms of the dynamics of family structure. Class differences in both kinship and friendship patterns have been well documented. Middle-class kin relationships are more geographically dispersed, but sustained over quite long distances through relatively close contact. Working class kinship ties are typically closer-knit, both geographically and in the intensity of the interaction among kin. The most striking class differences, however, are in friendship patterns. Despite the popular image of traditional working class communities as friendly, gregarious and warm, this is somewhat misleading from at least two points of view. Successive studies have shown that working class people have fewer friends than their middle class counterparts. And the contexts in which interaction with their friends takes place are more limited than in the case of middle-class people (Allan, 1985, pp. 71–2). A common explanation of this difference (and of differential class participation in voluntary organizations) is in terms of the greater social skills possessed by the middle class for forming and keeping friends in a variety of social settings, in part a result of greater middle-class career mobility.

A more convincing explanation may be in terms of the part which the home plays in developing and sustaining non-kin relations. Middle-class people typically foster friendships with new acquaintances by inviting them to, and entertaining them in, their own homes, thus broadening the relationship beyond the original setting in which they met. The relationship thus becomes, to some extent, an end in itself and not confined to a particular milieu, with the cachet that the friend is admitted into the private realm, the home.

Working-class people, on the other hand, do not use the home as a setting in which to develop friendships in the same way. Even important informal relationships tend to be compartmentalized in the contexts in which they first developed – work, common recreation, locality – and are not extended into the home.

Generally in working-class life, contrary to popular wisdom, the home tends to be defined as a private arena reserved principally for family members. Normally non-kin are not entertained in it, unless through some exceptional circumstance they have come to be regarded as almost 'honorary' family members. In this sense the working-class home can be viewed as something of a refuge from the outside world, a protected retreat into which unrelated others are not often invited (Allan, 1985, p. 72).

Even the tightly-knit informal networks of the traditional working class community did not rest upon friendship, but rather upon relationships between 'mates' (for men) and group sociability (for both men and women). 'Mate' relationships are different from friendship in that they are defined by the context in which the relationship develops – work, the pub, a common interest in football – and interaction is restricted to these specific contexts or linked to specific activities.

Group sociability is an extension of this type of relationship to several individuals. The archetype in the past was a group of men who both worked together and drank together in pub or club, but a variety of examples can be found. Their defining characteristic is that interaction is consequent upon joint participation in a particular setting. 'The group emerges from the setting and is largely confined to it' (Allan, 1979, p. 86). The group has an existence of its own over and above the people making it up. At earlier ages, juvenile gangs have some of the same characteristics (cf. Thrasher, 1928).

Generalizing these differences, Allan suggests that 'the rules of relevance which shape sociable relationships emphasise the personal relationship whatever the social setting in which it occurs for the middle class, but affirm the primacy of the interactional setting in which the relationship develops for the working class' (Allan, 1979, p. 83). This difference has considerable significance for personal ties and informal care. As noted, restricting access to the home among the working class means that home-based activities are confined to the nuclear and extended family. Where the contexts in which interaction with friends and mates occur alter, as a result of occupational change, urban renewal or long-range geographical mobility, informal ties with non-kin may be more likely to become attenuated, resulting in privatization. Moreover, in situations of dependency and need which would make informal care by non-kin one solution to providing care, there may be considerable resistance to admitting non-kin into the home. This issue will be returned to in Chapter 3.

The extent of privatization cannot be explained satisfactorily purely in terms of patterns of sociability among kin and non-kin. The contribution of successful working-class political struggles has brought about the attenuation of the mutual aid which was an integral part of communal solidarity.

> As long as workers were exposed to the precariousness of life governed by market forces, neighbourhoods and local communities provided some meagre collective self-defence by acting as units of self-help. . . . With the emergence of the welfare state, however, communal solidarity became less of a functional necessity so that neighbourhood communities have not been reconstituted, on the same basis . . . The achievement of the welfare state has thus tended toward a process of individuation, so that people come to exist as individual citizens in civil society, with home or family based collective social identities, rather than the class-based identities generated and sustained by traditional patterns of working-class culture and community. (Newby *et al.*, 1985, pp. 98–9)

Such identities may, for certain groups and classes, be more significant in mediating their political interests than work-based identities. Changes in the non-work sphere may thus form an important contribution to a decline in political involvement and a retreat into a privatized world within the home. In this situation, more transient contacts, what Clyde Mitchell (1966) has called categorical relationships, assume more importance. The prime example of this in British inner cities is inter-racial contact, often not based on personal ties but not taking place within an institutional framework, either. Where there is a lack of strong neighbourhood organizations, such primordial ties may assume considerable importance, particularly for members of ethnic minorities, as a way of providing care which goes beyond the family (Thomas, 1986, p. 109). Negatively, they appear in extreme form in phenomena such as racial attacks on minorities by members of the white majority.

MODERN COMMUNAL LIFE

The decline of communal solidarity and increase in privatization has clear implications for the significance of locality beyond the obvious point that the locality is no longer the centre of most people's lives in the way that it was in the past for some sections of the population.

> The spatial structure of the private social order is defined by two extremes of the metropolitan environment, the household, and the metropolitan-wide network of personal relations that link these private nodes. As Fischer (1977) and Wellman and Leighton (1979) have found in their recent research, the physical distribution of friendship is seldom constrained to physical proximity, as in the neighbourhood, but is widely distributed within the metropolitan field. . . . The metropolitan-wide spatial network of the private order is especially important for the mutual interaction between the private and the public orders (Hunter, 1985, p. 235).

It does not follow that the locality or neighbourhood are therefore not significant, rather, that instead of taking for granted the existence of local ties their creation has to be consciously worked at. Philip Abrams made the point trenchantly in relation to neighbourhood.

> Modern neighbourhoodism is in its purest forms an attempt by newcomers to *create* a local social world through political or quasi-political action. Great organisational skills and ingenious organisational devices are often used in attempts to mobilise old and new residents alike in order to protect amenities, enhance resources and, to a greater or lesser degree wrench control of the local milieu from outside authorities and vest it in strictly local hands. Much of the driving force and most of the

success of the enormous diversity of neighbourhood care projects up and down the country springs from these sources.
Traditional informal networks are dying and should be allowed
to die. Neighbourhood care today means working out a con-
structive relationship between the state, nationally and locally,
and neighbourhoodism, the politicised voice of local attachment. (Bulmer, 1986a, p. 95)

Sociologists since Toennies and Durkheim have grappled to
identify the sources of cohesion and solidarity in society. Industrialization swept away what Durkheim called the 'little aggrega-
tions' (including the neighbourhood) in which people existed in
the past and which were the centre of their lives. There was an
increasing polarization between the centralizing state on the one
hand and the mass of individuals on the other, moving formlessly
'like so many liquid molecules'.

The absence of all corporative institutions creates, in the
organisation of a people like ours, a void whose importance it is
difficult to exaggerate. . . . Where the state is the only environment in which men can live communal lives, they inevitably
lose contact, become detached, and thus society disintegrates.
A nation can be maintained only if, between the state and the
individual, there is intercalated a whole series of secondary
groups near enough to the individuals to attract them strongly
in their sphere of action and drag them in this way, into the
general torrent of social life (Durkheim, 1933, pp. 29 and 28).

A useful sociological attempt to bridge this gap, while recognizing the virtual disappearance of the traditional neighbourhood, is the concept of the community of limited liability
(Janowitz, 1952; Hunter and Suttles, 1972). In this conception,
community is seen as a mosaic of partially overlapping locally
based activities, groups and administrative areas. The citizen
participates in more than one community of limited liability and
has more than one partner or adversary in maintaining more than
one identity. 'Participation in the community of limited liability
is a voluntary choice among options rather than one prescribed on
the basis of residence alone. . . . Such a mosaic of overlapping
districts means that the loyalties, interests and demands of co-residents are quite fragmented because those who save them or act as

their advocates are equally fragmented' (Hunter and Suttles, 1972, pp. 59–60). Communities of limited liability tend to be a creation of administrative boundaries, perceived common interests, or shared residential fate (for example, an area affected by a planning decision). The expanding community of limited liability is a widening of this common basis for action to larger geographical areas such as a district or part of a town (cf. Hunter and Riger, 1986, pp. 63–4). The question of the geographical scale on which 'community' is supposed by policy-makers to exist is examined once more in Chapter 6.

More recently, Peter Berger (Berger, 1980; Berger and Neuhaus, 1977) has taken up this Durkheimian theme, contrasting the mega-structures of society – remote, impersonal and hard to understand – with private life, where meaning and identity are discovered and enjoyed. The relative lack of intermediate institutions not only leaves the individual vulnerable in time of crisis – as, for example, when in need of social care – but threatens the political order by depriving it of the moral foundations on which it rests. Berger argues that 'mediating structures' are required between the two extremes of society and private life to provide a focus for social activity and a point of attachment. It is not enough to foster unions of *gesellschaft* or pseudo-*gemeinschaft*. Structural provision must be made for people to develop secondary attachments.

Durkheim's well-known solution to this dilemma was to foster corporations (occupational associations), as a means of sustaining communal life without threatening the nation-state. In his view, geographical units such as the neighbourhood or local community lacked the potential to provide the basis for social action. Neither the locality, nor the department, nor the province had, in his view, enough influence to exert moral authority over the individual. 'It is impossible to artificially resuscitate a particularistic spirit which no longer has any foundation' (Durkheim, 1952, p. 390). Other sociologists are less sceptical, while recognizing that the concept of 'community' has outlived its usefulness. 'The question of how residential solidarities are keyed into other social arrangements bears on almost all the problems of societal integration' (Hunter and Suttles, 1972, p. 45). The neighbourhood or locality may play a politically and socially integrating role.

The issue has been faced most sharply in American discussions of the merits of 'local control', the attempt to restore to the very local level some degree of political involvement in decisions affecting the locality. Consider, for example, the claim that:

> there is special virtue of politics based on a small space, in which some people can, by and large, know one another and share some sense of the place in which they live – and consequently share civic interests. Politics in a space of human scale permits face-to-face citizenship (Morris and Hess, 1975, p. 9).

'Local control' refers to control at the neighbourhood, not city-wide, level; the British equivalent would be wards or parish councils, which have insignificant powers. The US National Commission on Neighborhoods suggested that:

> neighborhoods serve as important mediating structures between individuals in their private lives and the larger institutions of public life. Neighborhoods are the settings within which human scale organizations operate – the churches, schools, civic associations, and small businesses that serve to bring the individual into the social fabric of the community. By using the mediating structure of the neighborhood and its local institutions as channels for human services, they can be organized and delivered in ways that more adequately meet the needs of individuals. At the same time, residents can contribute their own strengths to the community by participating in the development of services (National Commission on Neighborhoods, 1979, pp. 234–5).

Reflecting upon the American debates about local control, Morris Janowitz and Gerald Suttles suggest that the locality provides a milieu in which the civic ideals of democracy can be given some meaning in face-to-face encounters.

> The survival of parliamentary democracies depends heavily upon how nearly its separate, local parts – its more intimate circles – relate to and interpret the larger movements of the wider society. Here, the local community seems to have a central, if not unique, role. Where the family, the peer group, and the church congregation tend to be very homogeneous and to have very narrow interests, the local community creates a

potential interface between diverse interests and the opportunity to debate, sort, sift and balance each against the other.
This potential is of extraordinary importance, for while it is the
habit of sociologists and most contrived groups to speak of
narrowly defined interests, real individuals are the repository
of an aggregate of interests, most of them poorly represented
by the formal groups that currently have an acknowledged role
in the political process. It is in the local community that individuals have the opportunity – by no means always realized –
both to internalize and aggregate the diverse gains and costs of
public policy (Janowitz and Suttles, 1978, pp. 84–5).

The import of this for 'community care' is that there are not
(contrary to what some policy-makers seem to believe) informal
social networks 'out there' waiting to be tapped. As this chapter
has argued, traditional locally based social networks are in
decline, and people's attachments are both more widely spread
geographically and also to some extent more privatized within
the nuclear family. Although both *gemeinschaftlich* and
gesellschaftlich relationships can coexist in the same milieu, of
greater significance for the fostering of local attachment is the
development of secondary structures for the fostering of local
attachment. Such mediating structures are not 'natural'; they have
to be created. Under whose auspices they are created, the composition of their leadership and membership, their objectives, all
have greater importance in determining their appeal and effectiveness at the local level. Such issues are almost entirely glossed
over in current debates about the provision of 'community care',
modulated moreover in a largely passive voice. Those who are
the object of care rarely get an opportunity to state their views,
still less organize for change.

NOTES

1   Classic studies have examined the Hawthorne bank-wiring room
(Roethlisberger and Dickson, 1939), combat groups in the US army
(Stouffer *et al.*, 1949), social cohesion in the *Wehrmacht* (Shils and
Janowitz, 1948) or informal processes in organizations such as the
police and welfare (Gouldner, 1954; Blau, 1963; Muir, 1977).

2   Considerable attention is given to patterns of neighbouring in Ruth

Glass's (1948) study of Middlesborough, Leo Kuper's (1953) frequently overlooked investigation in Coventry, John Mogey's (1956) comparison of two estates in Oxford and H. E. Bracey's (1964) comparison of new estates and subdivisions in England and America. A further comparative dimension is provided by Ronald Dore's study of neighbourly relations in a Tokyo ward (Dore, 1958, pp. 253–68). This and other literature is reviewed by Robinson and Abrams (1977) and Robinson and Robinson (1981).

3   Among historians whose work has embodied the idea he considers Bernard Bailyn, Gordon Wood, Oscar Handlin, Stephan Thernstrom, Stanley Elkins and Robert Wiebe. An example is provided by Wiebe's influential study *The Search for Order*, which argues that between 1880 and 1900, the United States moved from being a society based upon 'island communities' characterized by autonomy, informality and face-to-face relations to a centralized, formalized national society characterized by functional specialization and impersonality. Wiebe's monograph examines reform movements as responses to these trends (1967, pp. xiii-xiv).

3

Personal Ties in the Provision of Social Care

How is informal care provided and what scope is there for its expansion? These questions are considered in this chapter by looking at the personal ties on which informal care rests. Existing provision is briefly summarized, before looking at some of the obstacles to and difficulties in expanding 'community care' as a means of delivering welfare services to those in need. The main forms of informal care are well-known, and can be considered in terms of kinship, friendship and neighbourliness.

KINSHIP TIES

Kin ties remain the most important source of informal care for the majority of the population. 'Kinship continues to play a central role and at crucial stages in life remains the predominant source of care' (Willmott, 1986a, p. 28). Within the web of kinship relations, the nuclear family is central and the source of most caring relationships. Ties with extended kin are very much a matter of personal choice; those with members of one's nuclear family are more enduring and more likely to lead to responsibility for care.

Peter Willmott has documented some of the recent changes in

kin patterns. There are fewer elderly people living with children, siblings or other relatives, and a higher proportion living alone or just with their spouse. A study by Mark Abrams (1978) showed that one-third of elderly people had no living children. Among all elderly people, several studies have suggested that, of relatives seen, children comprise about half, brothers or sisters about a quarter, and more distant kin the remaining quarter. Between two-thirds and three-quarters of elderly people see at least one relative once a week, parent-child ties predominating over others.

As Willmott observes, kinship remains a major force in the lives of most people, and for those in need of care, provides the main source of helpers. This is despite a number of social changes over the last generation. These include the marked decrease in parents and adult children sharing a dwelling, with improvements in housing stock; greater geographical mobility, so that close kin no longer live within walking distance of each other; changes in men's and women's roles; increased divorce; and increased cohabitation without marriage. The resilience of kinship is to be found in the strength of the nuclear family – in ties between parents and their children, and between siblings – and by the spread of car ownership and the telephone, thereby enabling people to keep in touch. It is no longer necessary for kin to live in the same locality to keep in touch, and quite close contact may be maintained on a regular basis, over considerable distances.

Summing up the present situation, Willmott distinguishes four types of kinship system in contemporary Britain. He estimates that approximately one in eight of the population belong to a local extended family of the traditional type, such as those described by Dennis, Henriques and Slaughter (1956) in Featherstone, Young and Willmott (1957) in East London and Rosser and Harris (1965) in Swansea. Such a pattern is more common among the working class, in stable communities, and in the industrial north of England, Scotland and Wales. Approximately half the population belong to a dispersed extended family, which resembles the local extended family except that its base is not local and meetings are less frequent. The dispersed extended family is common among both the middle and working classes, and is critically dependent upon the motor car and the telephone. Aid and support, given in particular by married children to elderly parents, is provided

Table 3.1   *Sources of Help for People Aged 65 and Over, England 1976*

	Bathing	Cutting toe-nails	Going out-doors	Shopping (home-bound)
Percentage of those needing help who received it from:				
Person(s) in household	61	16	57	64
Relative(s) outside	19	5	28	21
Friend(s) outside	5	1	11	11
District nurse/health visitor	9	3	—	—
Home help	2	—	2	13
Chiropodist	—	73	—	—
Other person outside	4	1	5	4
No help received/not stated	4	4	17	3
Number needing help	473	747	243	150

Source: Willmott (1986a, p. 32), based on Rossiter and Wicks' (1982) adaptation of data from Hunt (1978). Percentages add to more than 100 per cent because some respondents mentioned more than one source of help.

© Policy Studies Institute 1986. Reproduced by permission.

regularly and in crisis situations. Contact is on a regular basis, perhaps once a week or once a fortnight.

A third type, Willmott suggests, is the dispersed kinship network. Contact among the nuclear family and with grandparents is maintained by phone and letter, with occasional visits across considerable distances, particularly at Christmas time. Members do not provide regular help for each other, but crisis assistance in childbirth or illness and, on occasion, financial help is provided, particularly among the middle class (cf. Bell, 1968). About one-third of the population belongs to such a network at any one time.

A fourth type is the residual kinship network, which includes perhaps one in twenty, or five per cent of the population, when some contact is maintained but relatives are rarely seen. As an arrangement for providing care, no kinship structure exists.

There is abundant evidence that members of the nuclear family are the key source of social care for the infirm and dependants. Data from a national survey form the basis of Table 3.1, which shows that three-fifths of elderly people needing help with shopping, going outdoors or bathing, receive such help from members of the same household (the vast majority of whom are kin) and a further one-fifth to one-quarter receive help from relatives resident elsewhere. No other source is of comparable importance apart from the specialist chiropody service. Only a minority of over-65s need help at any one time – the need increases markedly with age, particularly with the over-75s – and the first source of support is the spouse. Mutual help between married couples is a very important source of informal care and one that is insufficiently recognized (cf. Ungerson, 1983a,b). Married couples are also a critical source of psychological support. An American study by Hoyt and Babchuk (1983) showed that there was marked variation within kinship networks in who was likely to be chosen as an intimate or confidant. Spouses were about thirty times more likely to be selected as a confidant than an extended relative or a young child, about seven times as likely to be chosen as a parent, fifteen times as likely as a sibling, and ten times as likely as an adult child. For those aged 75 and over, these differences were much less, reflecting the greater degree of dependency.

As the support and care that is required gradually becomes more extensive with increasing age, the more likely it is to be provided by other relatives, principally daughters or daughters-in-law. Study after study attests to the crucial role such relatives play in sustaining the elderly and providing those who require it with assistance in such tasks as preparing food, shopping, laundering and toileting (Allan, 1985, p. 129).

Some of the care needed is psychological and material support, some actual tending, to revert to the distinctions suggested in Chapter 1. Visiting elderly people on a regular basis is different from doing their shopping, or cooking, or taking them out in the car, but these activities, in turn, are different from bathing, lifting, feeding or toileting. As an elderly person becomes more dependent, the care required can range from increased material support to different types and degrees of tending. The latter, in particular, may impose considerable strains upon the carers, both physically and emotionally. The growing policy interest in 'caring for the carers', particularly in cases where an elderly person is caring for his or her elderly spouse, is a reflection of this. More-over, as noted earlier, such care tends to devolve upon women. There are both social norms and taboos which make it appear that tending, in particular, is most 'naturally' provided by the wife for a married couple or the daughter for an elderly parent. 'The support at a daily level is almost wholly given by women and is defined as a development of their routine domestic role' (Allan, 1985, p. 130).

FRIENDS AND NEIGHBOURS

By comparison with kin, friends and neighbours are a much less significant source of informal social care and support. Friendships are usually made on the basis of common interest or experience, whether in childhood, in education, at work, in the pursuit of leisure, bringing up children or living in the same locality. One's friends are likely to be of a similar age and life stage and probably education and social status (Allan, 1979; Willmott, 1987). Friends are chosen, whereas relatives are given by the fact of the relation-ship. Friends are a source of reciprocal support, particularly for families with young children who may not have kin immediately nearby. Indeed, a notion of equivalency tends to be built into such relationships, the idea that each party is able to contribute equiv-alent financial and emotional resources to the relationship.

> The majority of routine mate and friendships are not par-ticularly well-suited for providing [informal] care. . . . While friends are likely to be concerned for each other's welfare, transforming this into long term active 'tending' is a different matter. . . . The basis of equivalency clearly breaks down when one side is unilaterally in need of and receiving care from the other. . . . The inherent imbalance such caring generates is ultimately likely to undermine the relationship's basis (Allan, 1983, p. 427).

A number of studies show that friends are relatively unimpor-tant as a source of social care, particularly in relation to 'tending' care (Willmott, 1986a, p. 71). The dependent elderly are ten times as likely to be helped by relatives as by friends. Friends may be of more importance than this suggests for psychological support

among the elderly, but in a sense this is a subsidiary contribution.
If basis 'tending' is not provided, the dependent person may not
be able to cope. If this 'tending' is provided informally, it is much
more likely to be provided by kin on the basis of permanent ties
entailing certain social obligations, than by friends with whom
the relationship has its origin in shared sociability. Thus, in Table
3.1 on p. 74, only one in twenty respondents received help with
bathing from friends outside the household.

Neighbourliness is a further source of informal support which
may assume importance for social care. Neighbours are those
with whom one lives in close residential proximity and with
whom one has face-to-face contact, if only passing each other in
the street. Neighbours are not chosen, and one only has a relationship so long as you and they continue to live in the same place.
Help between neighbours can be particularly useful in meeting
the contingencies of everyday life, minor help with letting people
into the house like meter readers or delivery men, keeping an eye
on things in holiday periods, visiting the elderly, or short-term
loan of minor items. In addition, neighbours can provide short-
term help in an emergency – such as a death in the family, or an
elderly person falling ill – until kin care or statutory care can be
arranged on a more continuing basis. There is some scope, particularly where the care of children is involved, for transforming
neighbourliness into friendship, but this is comparatively
unusual. There have been more sustained efforts to organize care
through so-called neighbourhood care schemes (Abrams *et al.*,
1981; Bulmer, 1986a), but although these have achieved some
success in providing visiting and transport services for the elderly
in a few areas, the national picture is patchy and generally provision of care is inversely related to the need for such care in a
particular area.

If kinship relations are based on obligation arising out of blood
ties, and friendship upon affective ties formed out of choice,
neighbourliness arises out of proximity. It is therefore all the
more necessary for social boundaries to be drawn to the relationship, and the ways in which this can be done will be discussed
shortly. A consequence of this, as Philip Abrams observed, is that
long-term, arduous, continuing care of an elderly or disabled
person would be most unlikely to be undertaken by a neighbour,
unless there were added to it some additional element such as

friendship. Neighbourliness is also in part a function of length of residence, so that the higher the rate of turnover of population, the less likely there is to be contact with neighbours. Again, like friendship, neighbourliness may be a source of psychological support and keeping an eye on the well-being of a dependent person. Neighbourliness can also be a means of alerting others if the dependency of the person increases (cf. Willmott, 1986a, pp. 59–60).

A useful way of looking at ties of kinship, friendship and neighbourliness is in terms of complementarity (cf. Litwak and Szelenyi, 1969). Different types of relationship may perform different functions. Kin ties are typically long-term ties, whether or not there is regular face-to-face contact with relatives. Ties with neighbours are face-to-face contacts and often time-urgent, as with borrowing small necessities or help in emergencies. Ties with friends have an affective basis reinforced by common interests or experience, and may or may not involve frequent face-to-face contacts. Given these different functions, it is not surprising that as sources of care, kin, friends and neighbours tend to meet different types of need, rather than substitute for one another, though some substitution, particularly in providing psychological support and domestic care, does take place.

> In consequence, despite substitution, people without available kin, particularly close kin, are less likely to receive informal care than those who have them. This applies particularly to elderly people; younger families seem to be more able to create networks among their peers which are adequate in meeting most of their day to day needs, partly perhaps because the help they need is less demanding and more easily reciprocated. (Willmott, 1986a, p. 74)

It is true that the distinctions may break down in practice. Philip Abrams was particularly interested in the potential for converting neighbourliness into friendship, and developed the argument at some length (Bulmer, 1986a, pp. 95–9). In an unpublished paper, he argued strongly that friends, neighbours and kin should not be seen as mutually exclusive:

> Attempts such as those of Keller (1968) and Schmalenbach (1961) to differentiate friends, neighbours and kin in principle

are persistently confounded by the creativeness of ordinary life. The most usual basis for such differentiations is that of constraint and choice. Thus, for Keller 'the neighbour is neither a relative nor a friend because the first is a prescribed relationship which one must acknowledge . . . and the second is a chosen one' (1968, p. 24). But in the real world kinship though perscribed is not entirely constrained; one may neglect, repudiate or even disinherit one's kin; conversely, the closest bond of kinship in many societies, that of marriage, is often engulfed in a dense ideology of free choice. On the other hand although friendship is chosen it is not entirely freely chosen; in practice friendship can be quite strongly constrained by settings, life-chances and the cost-reward balances of interaction. Neighbouring, for its part is also partly constrained and partly chosen; neighbours are there but can be ignored; they can be exploited or be-friended; they may make their presence felt but just how one feels it, and what one does about it, are open questions. Some transform neighbouring into friendship.

That transformation breaks down the conventional division of function between neighbouring and friendship and kinship so far as helping and social care are concerned. When neighbours become friends a relationship is re-constituted at a level of commitment and inclusiveness that makes it a powerful instrument of informal care. [It becomes] a relationship which has edged across a subtle barrier in terms of rewards, costs, trust and commitment.

There is also empirical evidence of such blurring of the lines. Laumann and Pappi (1966) found that 15 per cent of their respondents' friends were also kin. Townsend (1963) found a tendency to confuse neighbours and friends among his sample of the elderly.

Nevertheless, in terms of the basis of obligation to care, as argued in Chapter 5, kinship ties are qualitatively different from those with friends and neighbours. Too much emphasis *can* be placed on the obligatory character of kinship, but it remains true that as a source of long-term commitment, kinship ties are pre-eminent. Whether in the care of orphaned children or the dependent elderly, it tends to be kin who become the substitute parents or the carers in the majority of, though not in all, cases. There is a much lower probability of friends or neighbours assuming that role. Kin tend to be the first to be turned to.

From the point of view of community care policy, the most important questions concern the potential which non-kin primary groups have as carers, the ways in which non-kin relationships are interpreted and whether they can provide the basis for 'tending' care, and about the strain which caring imposes upon informal carers, whether non-kin or kin. In the remainder of this chapter, these questions will be examined in some detail in the context of isolation and loneliness among the elderly and privacy and revelation as a factor in relations between neighbours. A considerable proportion of the people in need of care of some kind receive this from their families, friends or neighbours, and are enabled to continue to live satisfactory lives in their own homes. Care policy must, given scarce resources, necessarily concentrate upon the more problematic and dependent cases of old age, disability, ill health and handicap. This means that the main client groups are the dependent elderly (particularly 75 and over) who suffer degrees of physical and/or mental impairment, who may or may not be housebound, the severely physically disabled who require assistance to perform daily tasks, the severely mentally ill, particularly discharged hospital patients diagnosed as psychotic, and both children and adults who are mentally handicapped.

Some of the social changes discussed in the previous chapter and at the beginning of this chapter mean that the kinds of social support available in the past from both kin and non-kin in stable, tightly-knit agricultural and industrial localities have been considerably diminished. 'Modern' neighbourhoodism, for instance, as Philip Abrams suggested, is much more a matter of mobility and choice within a more loosely knit network of personal ties (kin included). This, in turn, raises the question: What happens to those who fall through the net, who do not have social supporters who can help to maintain the dependent elderly, disabled or handicapped in their own homes?

THE ISOLATED AND LONELY

One way of answering the above question is by considering the situation of isolated and lonely elderly people, who are more likely, other things being equal, to be in need of formal and informal care in many situations. Since isolation and loneliness are a result of the attenuation of informal social ties, this is one way of understanding the determinants of lack of social support. A basic distinction may be made between social isolation, which is objective, and loneliness, which is subjective. Questions about the extent to which the individual interacts with others, and is part of wider social networks, can be answered objectively. How an individual feels – subjective states of loneliness, depression or happiness – are much more difficult to ascertain.

Discussing the condition of the elderly, four different types of social isolation have been distinguished (Shanas *et al.*, 1968, p. 260).

(1) *Peer-contrasted isolation*: comparing the isolated elderly with their contemporaries.
(2) *generation-contrasted isolation*: comparing the isolated elderly with younger people.
(3) *age-related isolation or desolation*: comparing the present situation of the isolated elderly with their social relationships and activities at an early stage in the life cycle.
(4) *preceding cohort isolation*: comparing the isolated elderly now with the preceding generation of old people.

Most research has focused upon the first type, while studies of bereavement among the elderly throw light on the third type of isolation.

An important distinction suggested by this typology and by other studies (e.g. Shanas *et al.*, 1968; Weiss, 1973a) is that between social isolation and emotional isolation (or desolation). Those who are *socially* isolated have relatively few social contacts and are not integrated into a large number of social networks. Those who are *emotionally* isolated may have a number of social contacts but lack an attachment figure (typically, among the elderly, due to death of the spouse) (Wenger, 1983, p. 148). It is an open question, to which we will return, of how far social isolation is a matter of choice. Certainly it may be to a greater extent than has sometimes been recognized. Emotional isolation, on the other hand, is usually not a matter of choice but of circumstance: the loss of a close emotional support due to bereavement, life-cycle change, geographical mobility or the ending of a relation-ship. Loneliness is clearly more subjective than isolation, being defined as an unwelcome feeling of lack or loss of companionship (cf. Shanas *et al.*, 1968, p. 269). Defining such a subjective state poses particular problems,[1] but clearly there is likely to be a close connection between emotional isolation and loneliness.

Problems of measuring isolation and loneliness will not be discussed here (see Wenger, 1983), but the meaning of isolation requires reconsideration in the light of dispersed kinship net-works and the existence of the telephone. The ability to keep in touch by telephone may make an elderly person more reliant upon distant kin, for example, than upon nearby neighbours or friends. The strength of ties in the geographically dispersed mid-dle class family is well documented from several British studies (Bell, 1968; Firth, Hubert and Forge, 1970; Allan, 1979). Such contacts are renewed from time to time face-to-face, but most regular contact is maintained by telephone.

Wellman's study in Toronto (1979, pp. 1211–14) found that one-third of respondents' intimate kin lived at some distance outside Metropolitan Toronto, ties with kin were the most actively maintained distant intimate ties, telephone contact was more frequent than face-to-face contact, and the two types of contact were complementary rather than substitutive. Fischer's study of friendship ties in Northern California showed that for the more important forms of interaction between friends – those involving the most intimacy, sacrifice and faith – people turned to intimates wherever they lived. Where the need was very great, distance was no object, because people came from far away. Moreover, more affluent respondents had more dispersed net-works and the constraints placed on their interaction by distance were weaker. In assessing the effects of geographical distance upon social isolation, attention needs to focus not only on the distances involved but upon the social class or socio-economic status of those involved. The barriers placed by distance on contact with kin are likely to be significantly greater for working-class than for middle-class people.

The main evidence about social isolation and loneliness comes from studies of the elderly. These show a relatively consistent picture of a small minority of the elderly suffering from high social isolation, corresponding to some extent to Willmott's residual kinship network, though there is not complete identity between those without close kin and those who are isolated. The most comprehensive cross-national study, by Shanas *et al.* (1968) showed that between two and three per cent of the elderly in Britain, Denmark and the United States lived alone, had had no visitors in the previous week, and had had no contact on the day prior to the interview. A much larger minority lived in semi-isolation. Around 15 per cent had seen no relatives at all in the previous week, and rather less than one quarter of respondents lived alone.[2]

Isolation, loneliness and lack of sociable contact, are therefore a minority phenomenon. The more interesting questions relate to determining the social characteristics and social conditions which lead to isolation and/or loneliness, which has bearing on the provision of care. The evidence is fairly clear, though not entirely conclusive.

There is an age-gradient for isolation and loneliness, the 'old' aged (persons age 75 and older) being more likely to lack sociable contacts. But age alone does not seem to be the explanatory variable, and Tornstam (1981) has shown that when other variables are controlled, age effects disappear. There are also marked differences between men and women. There are various factors to explain this difference, the principal one being the greater longevity of women and the greater likelihood of their having lost their partner.

Marital status also makes a difference. Wenger's data showed a marked difference on the loneliness measure between the married, and the single or widowed. In terms of self-perceived loneliness, however, the most marked difference was between the widowed and the single or married, the former being more lonely. Surprisingly, married women were more likely to be *very* lonely than any other group. This may be explained in part by the wife bearing anxieties and burdens as a result of her husband's poor health or anticipated death. It is also possible that relatives underestimate the social needs of elderly *couples* and visit them less (Wenger, 1984, p. 151).

'In addition to marital status, household living arrangements and family structure bear on the individual's likelihood of living in social isolation and being lonely. There is a strong correlation between the structure and density of an individual's immediate family network and his chances of living alone and in isolation' (Townsend and Tunstall, 1973, p. 248). Those living alone are particularly likely to be among the extremely isolated. Their isolation may, however, be reduced by social contact with relatives. A much higher proportion of the extremely isolated and partly isolated respondents in the Townsend and Tunstall study were childless, and a higher proportion had no relatives (3 per cent overall and 13 per cent among the extremely isolated). Thirty-seven per cent of the extremely isolated had seen no relatives in the previous week, compared to 13 per cent overall. Contact with kin was clearly a major form of social support.

Length of residence in the community appears to make a difference. Wenger's data shows that among the elderly who were age 40 or less when they came to live in the area, a smaller proportion reported self-perceived loneliness than among recent immigrants and a very small minority (4 per cent) scored 'high' on the loneliness measure. This finding may vary with types of area. Conflicting evidence is available about the extent of isolation in Inner London. Knight and Hayes (1981) found in a small sample a very high degree of isolation, and those who were isolated were very hostile to the area they lived in and identified crime and vandalism as the main causes of their dislike. Half of those interviewed only went out of their dwelling to work, or to shop or to go to the post office, and said they only mixed socially with members of their family. However, another small-scale study by Leat (1983a) in three localities showed more contact between neighbours, and higher degrees of neighbourly helping, in the Inner London estate studied than in two others, one in rural Kent.

Finally, state of health is clearly a factor, and one which is confounded particularly in the association between isolation and loneliness and age. Townsend and Tunstall (1973, p. 249) found a moderate association between personal incapacity and the likelihood of being partly or extremely isolated. Wenger shows a stronger association, those in fair or poor health showing a marked tendency to self-perceived loneliness and a high score on the loneliness measure, compared to those in excellent health.

This bare catalogue of influential factors is not sufficient to develop a theory of the causes of lack of social contact, but it

suggests some of the conditions which contribute to social isolation and loneliness. There is a need to complement data such as
those reported here from cross-sectional surveys with data on a
person's social networks. On the face of it, it seems likely that
those who are more isolated will be less integrated into wider
social networks. 'For the individual, the web of social contacts is
experienced as a whole, a network of social resources from within
which company, moral support, help and affection can be sought,
given and received' (Wenger, 1981, p. 75).

Wenger's data on support networks – including all those with
whom the respondent had close ties and from whom he or she
received regular help – suggest that small networks were most
common among single men, followed by widowed men. Almost
twice as many widowed as married men had small networks.
Slightly more of the single had small networks, while the married
were more likely to have large networks. There did appear to be
some relationship between network size and loneliness. No one
with a large network was often lonely, and more than twice as
many with small networks as with modal networks felt lonely
often. The networks of the single spread demands throughout the
network, while those of the married and widowed typically
concentrated on one significant other, either the spouse or one
child, respectively (Wenger, 1981, pp. 76–9). Differences in network size, though they may be related contingently to personality factors, cannot be explained away in that way, and are
shaped by social influences (Fischer and Phillips, 1982).

Social isolation is not caused by a single factor. Usually at least
three contributory conditions, and sometimes more, may be
present. This needs to be understood in framing community care
policies, for there are often no simple solutions to problems of
isolation. For example, daily visits from well-intentioned neighbours may not provide the right kind of support. Nor is it the
preserve of the elderly, who have been discussed here because of
availability of data. Loneliness among the elderly may, in fact, not
be particularly prevalent compared to others – those living alone,
college students, young mothers, the widowed, the divorced and
separated, recent migrants, and prisoners and their families
(Wenger, 1983, p. 146). One study (Lake, 1980) found that single
parents are the loneliest group. The situation of ex-patients from

mental illness and mental handicap hospitals has been little studied, but it is likely that as numbers in this category grow, isolation
and loneliness will be a particularly acute problem.

Certain factors and conditions may be picked out as of overriding importance in accounting for isolation and loneliness.

One is the intersection of familial and non-familial contacts.
Townsend and Tunstall (1973, p. 243) proposed a four-fold
typology relating kin ties and support to non-kin ties, each of
which could be strong or weak. Where both were weak, social
isolation resulted. Where family ties are weak, do other ties – with
neighbours, friends or other contacts (for example, a home help)
provide a (complete or partial) substitute? Where kinship ties
exist, to what extent do other ties complement or substitute for,
kinship ties? Here, of course, involvement with neighbours is of
particular interest, though relatively weak. There is, however,
evidence of the importance of friendship in socialization in old
age, acting as a buffer against isolation and loneliness (Jerrome,
1981, 1983; Cantor, 1979).

If the intersection of kinship with other types of sociable relations is the key to understanding social isolation, the key to
understanding emotional isolation and lack of support is loss of a
close significant other, in the elderly through bereavement. Much
of the most fruitful work related to isolation and loneliness has
arisen out of studies of bereavement (see especially Weiss, 1973a,
1982). Weiss, for example, suggests that the best way to learn
about the loneliness of emotional isolation is to study attachment.
To the extent that this form of loneliness is produced by the
absence of attachment figures, one should consider not so much
the variations in individual propensity toward loneliness as the
variations in the capacity for forming attachments and variations
in sensitivity to absences of attachment-providing relationships.
Similarly, research attention needs to be focused on social integration if we hope to understand the loneliness of social isolation
(Weiss, 1982, p. 78). (For an example see Wenger, 1982, pp.
221–5).

The association between depression and loneliness has been
established (cf. Brown and Harris, 1978), and a number of studies
of bereavement have highlighted the connection between loss and
loneliness.[3]

The Shanas study treated emotional isolation as 'desolation', typified by the loss through death, hospitalization or migration, of a social intimate, usually someone who is loved as a spouse or other close relative. Such desolation among the elderly is relatively high. The data which Shanas and colleagues gathered tended to support the hypothesis that desolation rather than peer-contrasted isolation was the causal antecedent of loneliness. 'Loneliness is related much more to "loss" than to enduring "isolation"' (Shanas, 1968, p. 276).

Several scholars have suggested the need to adopt a life course or biographical approach to the study of isolation and loneliness (Wenger, 1983, pp. 161–2). Elder and Rockwell (1979), for example, suggest that the stressfulness of change depends on (1) how drastic the change is (2) the individual's personal history (3) the stage in the life course at which the loss occurs. They consistently rank the death of a spouse as the highest magnitude of life change. How the elderly adapt, they suggest, can be predicted only in the context of their individual life histories. To take an obvious example, the social isolation of the elderly single person may not result in loneliness if that person has been single throughout his or her life and has successfully adapted to that state. Lowenthal and Haven (1968, p. 25) report that 'there are some life-long isolates and near-isolates whose later life adaptation apparently is not related to social resources'.

The earlier discussion of evidence on isolation and loneliness left open the relationship between the two. Does one lead to the other? Are they mutually independent? Or are they some way in between? Townsend's early study showed that those living in relative isolation from family and community did not always say they were lonely. Some people living at the centre of a large family complained of loneliness, and some living in extreme isolation emphasized that they were not lonely. Other evidence comes from data on what people do on Christmas Day. An American study (Benney *et al.*, 1959) showed that many of those spending Christmas in an apartment hotel did so by choice. A majority of the one-in-ten of Wenger's respondents who had not spent Christmas with family or friends did so by choice (Wenger, 1981, p. 42).

Townsend and Tunstall formulated the relationship negatively as follows:

Loneliness is not conditioned exclusively by physical or social segregation, or rather . . . it is not conditioned by contrasted isolation. In particular, people who are, by comparison with their peers, life-long isolates, are not usually lonely (Townsend and Tunstall, 1973, p. 259).

Wenger suggests that in looking at the very lonely among the elderly, friendship is more important than family contacts in determining loneliness. This may explain the lack of correlation with social isolation, which is usually measured predominantly in terms of family contacts.

It is clear that loneliness as a subjective state has very little to do with the actual amount of social contact. Some elderly people who have a high level of contact still feel lonely, while others who have little contact do not. The critical factor seems to be the state of health of the person involved. (Wenger, 1984, p. 174)

Wenger found that in her sample of 677 elderly people in North Wales, 1 per cent of those in good health, 5 per cent of those who described their health as all right for their age, and 13 per cent of those whose health was fair or poor saw themselves as being lonely often or most of the time (1984, p. 146). So long as health is good, those who are independent and with fewer social contacts appear not to feel lonely, but the situation changes with deteriorating health. There may also be difficulties in seeking help because of earlier social isolation, intensifying feelings of loneliness (Wenger, 1984, p. 174).

Loneliness may persist, even when frequent regular contact with family exists. Indeed, Wenger goes further and argues that 'the findings of researchers concerned with loneliness and morale have indicated that while family may provide instrumental support, friends assume a far greater importance where emotional and expressive backing is needed' (Wenger, 1983, p. 163). The policy conclusions drawn from this are particularly important for community care policies in general and neighbourliness in particular.

Much policy emphasis is placed on the role of the family. If old people are lonely, it is usually the family network which is seen to be at fault or lacking. Those who experience loneliness,

however, seem more likely to complain of lack of friendship –
and indeed friendship has been demonstrated to be more
important than familial support for morale and self-esteem.
Perhaps, therefore, caring professionals working with the
dependent elderly may need to pay additional attention to the
larger social networks of their clients, for whom friends may
prove to be the most important emotional resource (Wenger,
1983, p. 163).

Philip Abrams emphasized social choice as one of the factors,
together with mobility, leading to modern neighbourhoodism.
This perspective may be extended to isolation and loneliness to
suggest that inadequate attention has been paid to those who
choose to be socially isolated. Studies of dwellers in high-rise
apartments, for example, have suggested that people may avoid
others near whom they reside as a defence against crowding and
high density (Zito, 1974; McCarthy and Saegert, 1978). There are
hints at social isolation by choice in studies of the elderly, but it is
not fully developed (cf. Townsend, 1963, pp. 193–5). One group
which would be worth studying would be those who never
marry and remain single. Is this out of social choice, domestic
duty (for example, to aged parents) or what? The conditions
which may lead to isolation being a matter of choice can only be
sketched here, but they are undoubtedly important.

One general trend, implicit in Philip Abrams' concept of modern neighbourhoodism, though not spelled out, is the trend
toward privatization, discussed in Chapter 2. If the tendency to
concentrate upon the material well-being, social cohesiveness and
autonomy of the conjugal family is sustained, then wider kinship
and community ties would be likely to become more attenuated.
Sociability *within* the nuclear family would be stronger, but outside considerably weaker. To that extent people may choose a
degree of social isolation.

Further evidence of such a pattern is provided by the distinction
between the 'rough' and the 'respectable' working class (cf. Klein,
1965), which continues to crop up in local stratification studies.
Wallace, for example, in the Isle of Sheppey, found clear evidence
of such a divide on the working class estate studied, and a marked
tendency of the respectable to keep to themselves, to exercise

discretion, and to limit rather than extend social relationships (Wallace, 1984).

In turn, limits may be placed upon sociability by a sense of social superiority. The affluent upper middle-class manager or professional who moves to an isolated country location is one manifestation of this, but more interesting is the local resident who maintains social distance from neighbours on the grounds that they are social inferiors. Several such instances were found in the Abrams' team field studies (cf. Bulmer, 1986a, Chapter 4), and there are historical accounts (e.g. Roberts, 1971) which attest to this phenomenon in the past. Here are very clear cases of people who chose to be socially isolated, at least from their immediate neighbours, on grounds of social status. A concern with personal privacy, too, may lead to limiting social contact with others. Placing a social value on solitude, anonymity and reserve is likely to lead to a reduction in sociable contacts and to isolation, though not to loneliness (Derlega and Margulis, 1982, pp. 158–9). This is discussed further below.

Isolation and loneliness are thus complex social constructions. They are not immutable, and ties can be forged with the lonely to reduce their sense of being cut off from others. The care and sensitivity with which this needs to be done, however, has to be understood. For an elderly person suffering from emotional isolation (that is, desolation), providing social contacts of a superficial kind may be quite ineffective. Yet for that person to re-establish an intimate tie with another person may be a very difficult or impossible task, depending upon his or her age, personality and emotional resilience. It may be easier to provide material support and 'tending' than it is to provide effective psychological support.

PRIVACY AND SOCIAL CARE

Building community care upon informal social ties depends upon being able to open up channels of communication and assistance among non-kin, principally neighbours and friends. As noted above, however, people choose both with whom to have and whom not to have, contacts. It cannot be assumed by policy-makers that because potentially, in principle, social ties can be formed, that they actually will be formed. The clearest example of this is provided by ties between neighbours. What better way to combat loneliness and isolation, one might think, than to involve neighbours in breaking down the social isolation of the minority of the dependent elderly described earlier in the chapter? If only the warmth and communal helping of the traditional neighbourhood could be recaptured, the condition of the isolated elderly could be considerably ameliorated. It was emphasized, however, in Chapter 2, that traditional neighbourhoodism did not rest upon some 'natural' human tendency to be helpful, or on generalized goodwill to others, but was a specific response to economic adversity and deprivation, in which mutual aid was a way of coping. In the changed circumstances of the late twentieth century, with much greater overall prosperity, mobility and choice, such traditional patterns are unlikely to persist.

Such an approach also ignores the extent to which people build barriers as well as social ties between each other, particularly in situations of residential propinquity. In many situations where relative strangers are living cheek by jowl with each other, people are as concerned to maintain distance from each other as they are to foster close social ties. A powerful restraint upon the mobilization of informal social ties for caring is the desire to preserve personal privacy.

Privacy may be defined in terms of the control of information about oneself. It is 'the claim of individuals, groups or institutions to determine for themselves when, how and to what extent information is communicated to others' (Westin, 1970, p. 7). This implies that there will be some disclosure of information, and the individual who provides it should decide the nature and extent of such disclosure, or, indeed, whether to make the disclosure at all. Privacy is thus an interactional concept – it refers to the privacy of the individual or group vis-à-vis other individuals or groups, and to information transfer between them (Confidentiality, on the other hand, refers to the conditions under which such information, once communicated to another person, group or institution, is held, used and disclosed to third parties.) Discussion of privacy issues in the social welfare field have hitherto been almost entirely concerned with professional practices by doctors, social workers and others (cf. BASW, 1971; Hill, 1978; Wilson, 1978; Watson, 1985), and have paid little attention to ordinary people and the privacy implications of interaction between them.

Neighbours and Privacy

If one considers neighbours, it is well-established that most people look for the following qualities in a neighbour: friendliness, helpfulness and distance. Friendliness, which is very different from friendship, means easy and pleasant social intercourse of a superficial kind with those that one lives next to. A greeting between neighbours, for example, is usually both a turning toward but also a turning away. It implies good manners but also social distance between them (Pfiel, 1968, p. 147). Helpfulness means willingness to lend minor items for short periods, and to give more substantial help in crisis situations until other support can be mobilized. Distance means a recognition that being friendly and helpful does not mean that one has an intimate or close personal tie with one's neighbour. Maintaining one's own and other people's privacy is a positive social value and in some sense a social obligation (Bulmer, 1986a, pp. 28–31). The ideal neighbour is neither too interfering, too sociable nor too intimate.

These conclusions are based on several pieces of research. An early study by Leo Kuper in Coventry (1953) paid particular attention to privacy among neighbours. People in the area also distinguished between their neighbours, and were more reserved with some than with others. There was also differential sensitivity to the privacy needs of others among neighbours. There was wide variation in the practice of popping in and out of each other's houses. Some saw visiting as a threat to privacy, through neighbours getting to know your business, or as likely to breed familiarity, which, in turn, threatened privacy. The men visited other houses much less than the women. There was reluctance among both men and women to form friendships with neighbours. All of these findings suggest the fine gradations of proximity and distance, familiarity and reserve, through which local social relationships are conducted. H. E. Bracey's (1964) study of neighbours on new estates in Britain and the USA showed a similar concern with the preservation of privacy.

Referring to 'the guarded quality so characteristic of neighbouring', Philip Abrams (Bulmer, 1986a) emphasized the difference between friendliness – commonly cited as a characteristic of the good neighbour – and friendship. Friendliness is a desirable characteristic of casual interaction, involving a restricted conviviality which flourishes by carefully respecting each party's right to preserve the privacy of a 'back stage' realm. Friendship involves much deeper commitment, and involves progressively breaking down the barriers of privacy so essential to mere friendliness and steadily increasing the 'secrets' with which one is willing to trust the other. The longer a relationship is established the more likelihood there is of mutual confidence.

> Since a primary relationship involves the right of one person to invade the privacy of the other, most people will require some assurance that such a right will not be abused before entering into such a relationship. This assurance is gained through experience with the person. (Shulman, 1967)

Between neighbours, this barrier of reserve may never be broken down.

So far as neighbourliness was concerned, Abrams suggested that confidentiality was one of its cornerstones, and mutual respect for privacy the basis of tolerable neighbouring. It was put in an extreme form by the respondent who wrote a note to the interviewer: 'We don't want our neighbours talking about us so we're sorry we won't talk to you about them.' Such instinctive feelings about the boundaries between neighbours strongly suggest that reserve is an integral part of the relationship.

The 'Good Neighbour'

Several studies have elicited definitions of what people have meant by a 'good neighbour'. Kuper (1953, p. 64) obtained statements such as 'Don't believe in going into each other's houses', 'Keep themselves to themselves', 'Respects your privacy' and 'Not nosey'. A study of the social effects of planned rehousing by Vere Hole (1959) found a similar emphasis upon withdrawal and keeping one's neighbours at arm's length. A study by Kingston Polytechnic (1972) found a majority of both middle- and working-class respondents agreeing with the statement 'It doesn't pay to get too friendly with your neighbours' and a majority disagreeing with the statement 'A neighbour is someone you can tell your troubles to'. Colin and Mog Ball (1982)

suggested the need to strike a balance between privacy and open-
ness in neighbourliness. Philip Abrams's research elicited a large
number of responses reflecting this balance, and emphasizing the
resistance to unwanted intrusion. A large proportion of responses
referred to reserve or privacy – together with some alluding to
'nosey' or 'interfering' neighbours, or those 'always in and out'.
Typical definitions were:

> 'A good neighbour is someone who's friendly but not nosey
> and knows when not to come.'

> 'Someone who knows when they're wanted and when to
> disappear.'

> 'One you could call on but didn't live with you.'

> 'Someone friendly and helpful and who doesn't cause you any
> trouble, with noise and gossiping about you behind your back.'

> 'A good neighbour is someone who's always ready to help in a
> crisis but is not in and out of the house all the time.'

> 'A good neighbour is someone who respects your privacy and
> shows consideration.' (Bulmer, 1986a, pp. 53, 61, 66, 80.)

Policy discussion of the scope for involving neighbours in
informal social care tends to neglect the fact that neighbouring can
have negative as well as positive aspects, in which privacy concerns play an important part. Interpersonal conflicts, often over
trivial matters, can frequently arise between near or next door
neighbours. Parking, noise, smoke nuisance, or boundary issues
can all too easily become inflamed. As one Greenleigh respondent
told Young and Willmott (1962, p. 148), 'The policy here is don't
have a lot to do with each other [the neighbours] then there won't
be any trouble'. Recent studies of unemployment and the 'hidden
economy' found evidence that surveillance by neighbours was a
constraint on people's behaviour. Bell and McKee (1984) found
that the unemployed refrained from taking up certain outside
activities because they thought their neighbours would report
them to the DHSS. Wallace and Pahl's study of the Isle of Sheppey (1984; see also, Pahl, 1984) showed similar fears of being
reported to the DHSS by jealous neighbours, as well as at least
one case in which a local shopkeeper carefully watched the

amounts of money his unemployed customers had to spend so that he could report unusual affluence to the authorities. On relatively rare occasions, antagonism between social groups has become organized at the local level. Collison (1963) told the saga of the two estates in Oxford between which bad feeling reached such a high pitch that a wall was built between them – the Cutteslowe walls – to prevent contact.

Most contact between neighbours is much less dramatic than this, and does not involve elements of social control. As Mr Bennett remarks in *Pride and Prejudice*: 'For what do we live but to make sport of our neighbours, and to laugh at them in turn.' At a trial of a drug smuggling ring caught in Pembrokeshire due to the vigilance of local residents, prosecuting counsel observed that the accused forgot one thing, 'a characteristic you may think of rural life. Some call it neighbourliness, some call it over-curiosity, some would call it nosiness' (Bulmer, 1986a, p. 33). A desire to preserve one's privacy – to limit information about oneself and one's family known to neighbours – is a defence against that ubiquitous feature of local social intercourse: gossip.

Gossip

Gossip may be defined as informal personal talk about other people who are absent, about their conduct, and moral evaluation of that conduct (Bok, 1984, p. 91; Bailey, 1971, p. 288). As anthropologists and psychologists have shown (cf. Gluckman, 1963; Paine, 1967; Rosnow and Fine, 1976), gossip is a network of communication and a means of testing and reinforcing judgements about human nature. In another view, it is 'the more or less idle, more or less benevolent or malicious talk in which people engage in their efforts to construct a known and comfortable socio-spatial setting for their own lives' (Abrams, 1980, p. 18). It helps to assimilate and interpret bits of information about the lives of others. It bridges the gap between the private and the public worlds, and reduces reliance upon what people themselves wish to reveal. Gossip is a feature of informal personal networks linking kin, neighbours or friends.

Historically, gossip between and about neighbours has been a potent social force, both as a form of communication between neighbours and a means of social control. Robert Roberts describes how, in Edwardian Salford, the matriarchs in the working-class community in which he grew up guarded the collective conscience of the locality.

> From early morning to an hour before midnight, little groups . . . formed and faded, trading with goodwill, candour or cattishness the detailed gossip of a closed society. Over a period the health, honesty, conduct, history and connections of everyone in the neighbourhood would be examined. Each would be criticised, praised, censured openly or by hint and finally allotted by tacit consent a position on the social scale. (Roberts, 1973, p. 42).

Much of the talk was practical and useful, not merely malicious and scandal-mongering. But everyone's behaviour was minutely watched.

More recent studies by social scientists testify to the continuing importance of gossip. Despite the virtual disappearance of the traditional neighbourhood discussed in Chapter 2, Philip Abrams identified two contemporary survivals appertaining to this, close kinship relations between parents and children, and gossip. Kuper (1953) suggested that on the working-class council estate which he'studied, gossip was a means of sociability, a way of regulating status reputation and a form of social control, particularly through fear of what neighbours would say. A major reason for desiring privacy was to restrain gossip about oneself and one's intimates. Local residents emphasized that gossip could be malicious and improved in the telling, a source of local conflict, and a threat to privacy.

> Gossip is a notorious divider, the destroyer of privacy, that drags your life out from your private territory into the public forum. Many people we talked to had developed defences against the growth of gossip; there are useful lessons here for those working in neighbourhoods (Ball and Ball, 1982, p. 42).

Gossip is a touchstone of the ambivalent feelings neighbours can have about one another, involving friendliness and helpfulness on the one hand but distance and withdrawal on the other. Radcliffe-Brown suggested that where social relations are ambivalent, manifestations of social distance will be pronounced. This is certainly the case between neighbours, with a concern to defend one's privacy as a manifestation of the underlying ambivalence. The ambivalence recognizes the power which gossip, and the information upon which it is based, can possess. 'Neighbours are called upon in times of trouble; but they possess a lot of potentially dangerous information, and they are not inhibited in the use of this information to the same degree as kinsmen. Neighbours are thus a present help and a potential danger' (Heppenstall, 1971, p. 151).

There is also a rather fine line between more malicious types of gossip, rumour and scandal. This was well illustrated in one of the Abrams street studies by the case of a divorced woman on a new housing development who had cut off contact with her neighbours because of gossip about her. She did hairdressing at home, and because men came to have their hair cut at her home she was talked about. Her children were in care, her boyfriends became an object of interest, while her requests to husbands on the estate for lifts to work aroused jealousy in their wives. She commented:

> They're [the wives] all young and naive and don't know their own minds. Instead of staying at home and looking after their husbands and children, they go into each other's houses to gossip. And if they run short of talk one of them will knock on my door and ask to borrow something so that they can talk to me and try to find out what I'm doing (Bulmer, 1986a, p. 57).

Negative neighbouring and gossip may thus be quite closely connected.

The Private Realm as a World of Women

Women, in general, lead more locally based and domestic lives and are thus more likely to have the opportunity to engage in gossip. Indeed some feminists have pointed to the public/private dichotomy and maintain that it tends to equate with male/female, resulting in women being trapped within the domestic sphere (cf. Gamarnikow *et al.*, 1983, pp. 1–6). Since the vast majority of informal carers, as well as paid carers such as home helps and district nurses, are women, there is an important gender dimension to privacy (cf. Ungerson, 1987). The private realm, particularly so far as caring tasks are concerned, is a world of women.

This is not the place to enter into debates about broadening the public role of women and breaking down gender barriers, necessary though that task is. It is important to be clear, however, that the private, familial, sphere retains considerable social significance in bureaucratic, industrial society, as a sphere in which concern for others, responsibility, care and obligation are preferred values (cf. Gilligan, 1982).

> A world without the possibility for concealment, as the Nazi imperative had it 'without shadows', with no hiding places, nor refuge, nor solace, nor alternative to the force of the public sphere, is a world that invites barbarism or sterility or both (Elshtain, 1981, p. 335).

Issues of the gender basis of care are taken up again in Chapter 5, but the importance of this private realm for framing care policies needs to be borne in mind.

Privacy and Policy

Those policy-makers attempting to build informal care upon social ties between neighbours and friends need to consider some of the issues relating to privacy and gossip much more carefully than they have done hitherto. In particular, if the price for receiving informal care and support is likely to be the sharing of personal information about oneself with others, this may be deemed an unacceptable price to pay. This is most obvious in the case of those suffering from stigmatizing conditions such as alcoholism or mental illness, but it may also apply in different ways to recipients of Supplementary Benefit, to single mothers, or to families with a member who is mentally handicapped. Yet such people are members of precisely the client groups upon whom 'community care' is targetted. (The dependent elderly constitute the main other group.) Some of these issues are considered further in Chapter 6, but brief further consideration may be given here.

The Barclay Report (1982), for example, makes much play of the possibilities for 'interweaving' formal, statutory services with informal social support networks (networks are discussed further in the next chapter). How this may impinge upon the client has not been thought through.

Consider the exchange of information in caring arrangements

involving three parties, the person cared for, the welfare staff of a statutory agency (such as a local authority), and other members of the public with whom the person cared for shares membership of a common primary group and who are potentially available to provide informal care. The exchanges involved may be of four types: (1) between the person cared for and an agency staff member; (2) between the person cared for and a relation or a friend or a neighbour, without the agency staff member being involved; (3) between the agency staff member and a relation, or a friend or a neighbour of the client, without the person cared for being involved, and (4) between all three parties, with the knowledge and involvement of all three. While the first clearly falls within the realm of formal care, and the second within the sphere of informal care, the third and fourth fall in between (or in *both* public and private spheres). Issues of privacy and confidentiality are of particular salience in relation to such 'interweaving' of formal and informal care, yet they appear to have received little attention. Much closer consideration is needed of the circumstances under which information is shared under the third and fourth type, and the principles which should govern such exchanges. For example, is it permissible for welfare staff to exchange information with actual or potential informal carers about a client, without the informed consent of the client to the release of that information? Such a question is particularly pertinent in the case of conditions such as alcoholism or mental illness which are highly stigmatizing. To what extent, regardless of their condition, do people want personal information about themselves released to others?

There are also issues of public policy and political philosophy involved (cf. Bulmer, 1986d). In his strong dissent to the Barclay Report, Robert Pinker suggested that stimulating a flow of information about local needs into neighbourhood social services offices as part of community social work would lead to the proliferation of local data banks based largely on hearsay, gossip and well-meaning, but uninvited, prying. A key role was envisaged for those such as publicans, corner shop-keepers and school crossing attendants, well placed to gather such information.

It is important that some rapport exists between the formal and informal systems of social care. It is equally important that the state is not allowed to intrude too far into the private worlds of individuals, families and local communities (Barclay, 1982, p. 256).

Proponents of community social work have argued that the desire to protect privacy is exaggerated. It may, for example, be confined mainly to the middle classes. David Thomas (1986, p. 10) has argued that 'the only way to enjoy a private life for those who could not escape the inner cities was to be more active in getting to know, and working with, those around them'. The primary task of community workers should be to promote membership of people in locally based networks and groups which can overcome this isolation and privatization. There are genuine differences in interpretation here over why such isolation exists, but there are also analytic and normative weaknesses in a community work approach. The community or neighbourhood is hypothesized as a basis for attachments instead of the degree of people's local attachments being regarded as an empirical question. And the fostering of local activities is seen as a good thing. Those advocating such policies do not appear to have grasped the extent to which such policies may be perceived by those for whom they are intended as a threat to privacy. (For one example of complete avoidance of the issue, see Thomas, 1985.)

Privacy and Privatization

Is there a link between trends toward privatization – discussed in the previous chapter – and a desire for personal privacy? Privatization is a trend at the societal level, encouraged by greater affluence, better housing, consumerism, car ownership, and the telephone. Its study is a part of macro-sociology, commonly studied in relation to social stratification (e.g. Marshall *et al.*, 1985). The desire to protect one's personal activities from the scrutiny of others is a micro-phenomenon, concerned with social interaction and its management. There is thus a gap between the macro and micro levels, and the two need not necessarily fit together. Gossip, for example, is a phenomenon of all primary group relations in societies at different stages of social development, and there is no sign of its disappearance in contemporary urban society. Yet there is a connection between the macro and micro levels. Greater withdrawal into the home and lesser involvement in local communal activities reduces the opportunities for mutual scrutiny and observation of others.

In Salford at the turn of the century, Robert Roberts' parents in their corner shop could monitor closely their customers' financial status and make on-the-spot decisions as to whether to grant credit (Roberts, 1978). In the large urban shopping centre of today, filled with supermarkets, department stores and chain shops, many of them offering easily available credit to shoppers, there are much fewer face-to-face contacts between people known to each other. Financial worth is judged by possessing cheque cards or credit cards, or being a 'good risk' for a credit agreement. These financial transactions, in turn, require the citizen to deal with large financial bureaucracies to whom they have to reveal financial information about themselves, with consequent implications for privacy (cf. Rule 1973). In terms of local interaction, however, the individual has rather more personal privacy about his financial affairs. In the realm of care, this transition has been marked by the decline of locally based networks of kin and neighbours to provide support, and a greater reliance upon statutory helpers from the personal social service and health fields such as home helps and district nurses.

THE DIVERSITY OF CARE

This change is reflected in Willmott's classification of kinship systems mentioned earlier. The dispersed extended family and the dispersed kinship network are no longer based in a particular locality, yet they are much more characteristic of modern urban society than the rural village or the close-knit traditional industrial community. This loosening of network ties – considered further in the next chapter – has probably led to an increase in individuals' sense of personal privacy, but has also sharpened the possibilities for the exchange of information in the course of providing care. This is reflected in the wider range of types of care available today than in the early twentieth century. Formerly, care was principally available from informal carers, from voluntary organizations (of a charitable and usually marked social class in character, whether of aristocratic beneficence or working-class self-help), or from statutory sources, notably poor relief and the workhouse.

Today, at least seven different sources of care may be distinguished. (1) Informal care remains important, if not so tightly tied to the neighbourhood. (2) Self-help groups of an informal kind are another form of care, exemplified by Gingerbread for single parents and Mencap for parents with mentally handicapped children. The Association of Carers, which seeks to represent those who bear caring burdens at home, also falls into this category (cf. Briggs and Oliver, 1985). Voluntary activity falls into two types. (3) Locally based neighbourhood care schemes (cf. Abrams *et al.*, 1981) have only a loose and vestigial organization and aim to draw upon people living in the same area as those they care for. (4) More formal voluntary organizations, such as WRVS and Help the Aged, are, if not the direct descendant of Victorian philanthropy, organized on a national basis with local branches and a more substantial bureaucratic presence. In this category would also be included caring organizations with a religious basis, such as the Salvation Army and Dr Barnardo's. (5) Formal face-to-face social care is provided by statutory health and social services. This type of care has expanded enormously in the second half of the twentieth century, and is now the main source of help for those without close personal ties, as well as for many with such ties. (6) A further type of care is that provided impersonally, at a distance, through telephone advice services, of which Samaritans is the best known. (7) The last type is the private, commercial provision of care. This is most common for those at each end of the age range, and includes child-minding for the young (cf. Jackson and Jackson, 1979) and the provision of old people's homes for the dependent elderly. The latter have been a considerable growth area in Britain in recent years.

There has thus been a diversification of care during the present century, with recognition that a wider range of need and dependency can be met from different sources. One consequence of this has been that the sharing of information about the cared for has become more widespread and more formalized, with more opportunities for invasion of personal privacy. To be sure, early twentieth century industrial workers who were the object of upper-class beneficence (whether from their employer's family or elsewhere) enjoyed little personal privacy, but this was usually on the basis of some type of paternalistic relationship in which affective ties played a part. (These ties could be negative as well as positive, as sociological studies of deference have suggested.) Modern 'interweaving' of formal and informal care, discussed in Chapter 6, is constructed on the basis of generalized, human-itarian sentiments, that the needs of the dependent should be met, rather than upon personal ties. Indeed, policies of 'interweaving' seek to construct such ties, even when they do not exist, from such sentiments. The likelihood of infringements upon people's privacy is accordingly increased by such attempts at social engineering.

Trends toward privatization could also have implications for isolation and loneliness as social problems, but in this respect the dispersion of kinship networks is of much more significance. Moreover, there is a good deal of evidence, in relation to loneli-ness in particular, that it is not only the number and frequency of contacts that a person has but the quality of those contacts. Those involved in the planning of social care need to recognize that it is not just the existence of informal ties which is significant, but the basis of the attachment formed through the tie.

THE DECLINE OF COMMUNITY?

What of the validity of the Simmel–Wirth view of urban society as producing the rootless, unattached, isolate, consequent upon the collapse of community (see p. 44)? This is an issue of considerable policy importance, since one critique of the term 'community care' maintains that it does not refer to a useful abstraction. The Simmel–Wirth theory fits closely with theories of mass society which postulate the disorganizing effects of industrialization and bureaucratization upon the individual's attachment to primary groups. According to the 'community lost' theory, such ties are particularly likely to become attenuated in urban areas. This view does not find very convincing empirical support. Family ties seem, judging from a number of studies, to be as close and as psychologically important in the city as in the countryside. Peo-ple living in cities draw on the same types of support from different sources – kin, neighbours and friends – as they would in rural areas. For example, urban dwellers have just as many friends as those living in rural areas and seem to be able to form friendships quite quickly (Franck, 1980). Urban residents are involved in personal networks linking members of primary groups just as much as rural dwellers. To the extent that there are differences, the personal networks of urban dwellers are more widely spread geographically, and there is a slightly greater degree of specialization of function (Fischer, 1976, pp. 125–51). A comparison in Northern California of small-town and city respondents showed that they had roughly equally supportive social networks. 'The thesis that urban residents lack adequate social support finds little empirical support' (Fischer, 1982, p. 138). Though city dwellers had fewer people to look after their homes when away or to help in the house, people in small towns scored lower on counselling and companionship.

The thesis of what Wellman terms 'community lost' thus finds relatively little empirical support in the terms that Simmel and Wirth originally adumbrated it (Wellman, 1979, pp. 1223–4). Whether the converse, that is, the 'community saved' theory, holds, is also doubtful. Originally generated on the basis of studies such as Young and Willmott (1957) and Gans (1962) of the existence of 'urban villages' with solidary social ties, linked to territorial cohesiveness, this suggests that the prime allegiance of urban dwellers is to sets of relationships framed within particular neighbourhoods. Again, empirical evidence does not bear this out. In Willmott's kin classification quoted earlier, for example, he estimated that five-sixths of the British population have dispersed rather than existing locally concentrated kin ties (though some of this dispersion may be to a relatively short distance only). Studies of urban communities have documented the density of residents' local networks within the neighbourhood (cf. Suttles, 1968; Stack, 1974; Gans, 1967), but have not provided a picture of the total network of individuals resident in the locality. When this is done, the salience of the locality declines. Even helpful ideas such as the 'community of limited liability' (cf. Janowitz, 1952) have treated external linkages as spreading outwards from a local base in the neighbourhood, and have not provided a picture of weaker, sparsely-knit and dispersed ties which individuals form in urban and, increasingly, in rural areas in industrial society.

An alternative theory of modern urbanism, and one which is

Table 3.2   *A Comparison of the Community Lost, Community Saved and Community Liberated Theories, with Findings from a Study of East York, Toronto*

Argument	Community lost	Community saved	Community liberated	East York findings (main tendencies)
Basis of intimacy:				
Availability	Rare	Abundant	Abundant	5+ intimates
Relational	Formal role	Kin, neighbor-hood	Friendship, work	Kin, friendship
Spatial	Local	Local	Metro-politan, national	Metropolitan
Mode of contact	In person	In person	In person, telephone	Telephone, in person
Communal structure:				
Density	Sparse	Dense	Sparse	Sparse
Reciprocity	No	Yes	Uneven	Uneven
Boundedness	Ramified	Tight	Ramified	Ramified
Basis of assistance:				
Prevalence	Minimal	Abundant	Moderate	Moderate
Relational source	Formal ties	Kin, neighbor-hood	Friendship, work	Parent/child, work
Residential basis	Local*	Local	Metro-politan, national	Metropolitan
Density	Dense*	Dense	Sparse	N.S.
Structural source	Secondary	Solidary group	Network ties	Network ties

*To the extent to which primary ties exist.
Source: Wellman, 1979, p. 1224.
© 1979 by the University of Chicago. Reproduced by permission of the University of Chicago Press.

particularly pertinent to the study of social support, is what has been termed 'community liberated' (Wellman, 1979). In this view, ties between members of prime groups tend to form sparsely-knit, spatially-dispersed, extending networks instead of being bound up within a single densely-knit solidarity. Although kinship work and residence are not combined, such primary ties are important sources of sociability and support. The theory frees the concept of community from its purely local roots and allows for informal ties in terms of social networks.

> These networks, by their very nature, are not 'institutionally complete', self-contained 'urban villages'. Their sparsely-knit ramifying structures provide a broad range of direct and indirect connections to the dispersed and differentiated resources of industrial bureaucratic social systems. Obtaining resources through such a sparsely-knit network is not a matter of obligations due a member of a solidarity. Instead, it is a matter of the quality of the particular dyadic ties, the ease of maintaining contact, the ability of network members to provide indirect connections to additional resources, the extent to which additional members of a network can be mobilized to provide assistance, and the connectivity between networks (Wellman, 1979, p. 1207).

The main features of the 'community liberated' theory are presented in Table 3.2 and are contrasted with the theories of 'community lost' and 'community saved' and salient findings from Wellman's own study in East York, Toronto. As a starting point for the contemporary understanding of social support and 'community care', the 'community liberated' theory has much to commend it, both in reflecting twentieth-century social changes (particularly in use of the motor car and the telephone) and in providing a picture of modern urbanism more in accordance with empirical evidence. Use of the theory does, however, require close familiarity with social network analysis, and to this we turn in the next chapter.

NOTES

1   Lopata favours a rather more general definition than Shanas: 'loneliness is a sentiment felt by a person when he defines his experienced level or form of interaction as inadequate' (1969, p. 249). Tunstall (1968) favoured an operational definition: 'an old person is lonely if he says he feels lonely, and not otherwise'. A number of those writing about loneliness (e.g. Sheldon, 1948; Blau, 1973; M. Abrams, 1978) do not define the term at all, taking the meaning for granted (Wenger, 1983, p. 149).

2   In terms of self-perceived loneliness, 7 per cent described themselves

as lonely often or most of the time, 21 per cent as sometimes lonely and 72 per cent as never or rarely lonely (Shanas *et al.*, 1968, p. 271). This compares with responses to Wenger's similar question (N=683) which showed 5 per cent as lonely often or most of the time, 19 per cent as sometimes lonely and 76 per cent as never or rarely lonely. However, her eight-point loneliness measure classified 9 per cent as high (that is, very lonely), 29 per cent as medium and 63 per cent as low, suggesting that self-perceived loneliness may lead to under-estimation (Wenger, 1983, pp. 153–6).

3 Lopata (1969), for example, provides a very full classification, distinguishing between loneliness at missing the presence of other (spouse); as feeling no longer loved by the other; as missing the other as a love object; as lacking someone with whom to share experiences; as lacking someone with whom to share household tasks; as lacking the ability to make friends, and so on.

4

Personal Ties and Social Networks of Care

'Community care' is concerned with the resources available outside formal institutional structures, particularly in the informal relationships of the family, friends and neighbours, as a means of providing care. Yet as shown in Chapter 2, 'community' is hardly a satisfactory term to convey the social basis of such care. No longer is its provision geographically confined to particular localities, however much this was so in the past. Some means is needed, all the same, to refer to the personal ties between those involved in informal relationships of one kind or another. The term 'social network' has come to be used extensively, as a means of relating abstract concepts such as institution or group to the activities and relations of actual people.

The concept of social network is particularly useful for the analysis and understanding of local level informal social ties, of what Clyde Mitchell in an early influential paper distinguished as personal relationships (1966, pp. 54–6). He contrasted these personal ties to institutionalized relationships at work, in a political party, a church, and so on, and to categorical relationships, as when members of different races (his examples were drawn from Southern Africa) met in the market place and treated each other on the basis of perceived skin colour. Personal relationships are at the heart of informal care, but they are also a mainstay of local social relationships. The value of the term network lies in avoiding the reification involved in talking about 'community', yet enabling one to talk about a wider set of informal relationships than just the family or the extended kin group. The set of relationships has broadened to include friends, neighbours and work associates. There has always been an analytical problem for the social scientist to find a means of portraying such relationships. 'Social network' seems to be a useful way of doing so.

'Community care', however, is a practical policy, not just a matter for detached academic debate. The pursuit of the policy has been hampered by confusing terminology, pre-eminently in the term 'community' itself. To what extent do 'social network' and associated terms such as 'social support' provide a way round these problems? This chapter examines some of these issues in the application of network analysis, and begins by looking at some instances of such use in the field of social welfare policy. This is a prelude to tracing the origins of the approach in social anthropology, and teasing out some of the analytic insights which it can provide. Examples of applications in social welfare show that ideas of 'social network' and 'social support' have been taken up with enthusiasm, particularly but not exclusively in North America, so much so as to constitute what one recent observer has called 'a kind of romantic ideology for social work practice' (Specht, 1986, p. 219). Such uses in social welfare pose considerable problems, as the material later in the chapter will demonstrate.

SOCIAL NETWORKS IN COMMUNITY CARE

In discussions of provision of care and service delivery, the concept of 'social network' has come to be widely used. In Britain, the key source has been the Barclay Report on social work, published in 1982. Barclay defines 'community' as made up of 'local networks of formal and informal relationships, together with their capacity to mobilise individual and collective responses to adversity' (p. xiii). The majority of people in trouble turn first to their own families for support. If this is lacking or insufficient, people turn to wider kin, friends or neighbours, because seeking help from such informal networks is socially acceptable and seen as less of a blow than approaching officialdom. Thus help from kin, friends and neighbours is referred to as provided by informal caring networks, usually locally based.

Such usage is an application of the terminology by now common in anthropology and sociology, but it then takes on a life of its own. The Barclay Report recognized that informal networks are complex and not always benign. If links are made between informal and formal care, formal carers need to develop detailed knowledge of informal networks and work in close understanding with them. Partnerships need to be developed between formal and informal carers. 'Caring networks in a community need to have ready access to statutory and voluntary services and to contribute their experience to decisions on how resources contributed by these services are used within their community' (Barclay Report, 1982, p. 202). The majority of social care in Britain is provided not by statutory or voluntary agencies but by individual citizens who are often linked into informal caring networks. These informal carers, Barclay argued, need to be brought within the ambit of professional care.

Applied to social work, this meant that, although individuals or families with problems remained the centre of attention, the focus should be upon individuals within the networks of which they formed a part. 'The circle of vision is extended to include those who form, or might form, a social network into which the client is meshed. Social workers have to be able to take account of a variety of different kinds of network. These will vary in size and in the bonds which hold them together' (Barclay Report, 1982, p. 205). The social worker could make use of these networks in three ways. The first is the most obvious, moving out from an individual to the kin, friends and neighbours who constitute that person's network, to identify and map the most significant personalities in a client's life. Secondly, social workers could identify and build on the ties between those in a neighbourhood, residential home, day centre or hospital, to develop networks among people who live or spend time together. Thirdly, there was scope for developing networks among those sharing similar communities of interest or concern, for example, parents of mentally handicapped children.

The Barclay Report considered that a change was also needed in the orientation and role of social workers. What was pre-eminently required was an attitude of partnership.

> Clients, relations, neighbours and volunteers become partners with the social worker in developing and providing social care networks. We have already referred to the description of the relationship by one respondent as 'equal but different'; we might be prepared to go further and describe social workers as upholders of networks. This may make clear our view that the function of social workers is to enable, empower, support and encourage, but not usually to take over from, social networks (Barclay Report, 1982, p. 209).

In its advocacy of community social work, Barclay was thus placing great reliance upon the notion of network and its potential for harnessing to community care. In doing so, it reflected earlier American enthusiasm for the potential of networks in promoting social care. An early paper was Collins and Pancoast's *Natural Helping Networks* (1976), which argued that natural helping networks had tremendous potential in social welfare.

> They exist as semi-permanent social structures in all cultures, in cities as well as villages, among people of every class. Their importance for social order and integration may increase rather than diminish as society becomes more complex. Networks are one of the most vital bridges between the individual and the environment. Helping networks are the informal counterpart to organized social services, and in many areas carry the largest part of the service load (Collins and Pancoast, 1976, pp. 28–9).

Collins and Pancoast's focus was upon mutual aid, particularly among neighbours, and they saw what they called 'natural networks' as one of the key means of social support, absorbing the load which formal services could not cope with. Various techniques were suggested for harnessing these networks, one of the most important of which was the identification of what Collins and Pancoast called 'central figures' or 'natural neighbours' in a locality. 'Central figures' possess sufficient psychic resources to be on top of their own life situations to be able to give to others and respond to the needs of others. Some may establish that role purely on the basis of informal personal ties – for example, the

home-centred housewife who establishes links with other mothers and needy neighbours in the locality. Another way in which
such nodal figures may emerge is through a particular occupational role – for example, local shopkeepers, meter readers for
public utilities, local hairdressers and bar staff.

It is then suggested that social workers involved in neighbourhoods should seek to recruit such 'natural neighbours', through
whom the social worker could work in the locality to draw on
existing informal networks and extend them as a means of support. 'Central figures' would be encouraged to enlarge their social
circle to increase the effectiveness of the social network used to
provide informal care. This would bring in others previously
unknown either to professionals working locally or to the 'central
figure', both through personal efforts and referrals from other
professionals, alongside whom the 'central figure' works. Social
workers may refer other professionals to the 'central figure' to
effect such introductions. Though the 'central figure' remains
part of the informal system, the social worker recruiting such a
person must be satisfied as to his or her competence and responsibility, for example in respecting the confidentiality of information acquired in the course of the work. In *Natural Helping
Networks* both the notion of a network and the position of an
individual at a key position in such a network assume central
significance.

Such an approach to the analysis of informal care was taken
further in work by Charles Froland and others at the Regional
Research Institute for Human Services in Portland, Oregon.
Their work uses the term 'helping network' more broadly

> to describe a wide range of informal helping activities that staff
> in the agencies we studied have sought to identify, support and
> reinforce. . . . Emphasizing informal helping within the con-
> text of a *network* of relationships has distinct conceptual advan-
> tages to more traditional ways of viewing social relationships.
> The concept of network in its most general form draws our
> attention to the *structure* of relationships among a set of actors as
> well as the specific *exchanges* which take place among them and
> the *roles* they play with each other. Networks describe social
> relationships in fairly concrete terms. . . . Even the most
> socially isolated individuals and the most anomic communities

seem to have a few relationships of this sort. We all use our networks when we need information or special assistance. In turn, our networks influence us by channeling and shaping the kinds of information we take in. They also require certain forms of reciprocation as well as the ongoing effort of maintaining the linkages. Networks are part of a sense of who we are (Froland *et al*, 1981, pp. 19–20).

In an analysis of the work of social welfare agencies in providing social support through building upon networks, they identify five different strategies which may be followed. (1) A *personal networks* strategy is used by a professional worker to build upon the client's personal ties with kin, friends and neighbours, involving these significant others in the client's problems and their resolution. In some circumstances, attempts may be made to expand the client's range of social ties and support. (2) A *volunteer linking* strategy, on the other hand, may be invoked in situations where there is limited personal support. Here, an attempt is made to match the client with volunteer supporters, not previously known to him or her, who have had personal experience of the problem the client faces or who are willing to provide help. For example, help for the physically disabled was provided in one scheme by recruiting people who could advise upon the problems of independent living in the community.

(3) *Mutual aid networks*, as a third type, aim to build peer support by bringing together people who have experienced similar problems or have common interests. Similar in aim to self-help organizations, they are, however, informal without a charter or formal programme. Such networks may sustain existing efforts, develop new sources of support, or, in some circumstances, serve an advocacy role. Such networks can be used to promote a sense of normalization and social integration among clients such as ex-mental patients, and in them members may give and derive support without feelings of stigma or dependency.

The last two types of network build upon geographical propinquity. (4) In *neighbourhood helping networks* agencies they seek to identify and form relationships based upon existing local networks among neighbours, key figures, and local influential people such as clergy. Their aim is to help isolated individuals,

promote local mutual aid, identify local issues and promote informal social organization, often with particular client groups in
mind such as the housebound elderly, the disabled or discharged
mental patients. Consultative relationships are established to
work with neighbours to identify problems, and to encourage
local residents to become involved in helping activities. It is in this
type of network that the role of 'central figure' or 'natural neighbour' is most salient. It is claimed that 'staff may effectively reach
an entire community through a manageable number of individuals who are central linking and referral agents within the informal
social organisation of a community' (Froland *et al*, 1981, p. 79).

Finally, (5) *community empowerment networks* aim to establish
local action groups to meet local needs and provide community
forums through which local opinion may be articulated and
represented to policy-makers. Such an emphasis is more directly
political, and involves working with neighbourhood leaders
(who are not necessarily or even usually 'central figures' in informal networks), with local voluntary associations, and with
opinion leaders in local business, trade unions and churches. An
example is given of an agency who used such a strategy in an inner
city Polish Catholic working-class neighbourhood to seek better
mental health services. The aim is both to articulate the need for
formal services and to show how they could, if provided, be
integrated with the informal network existing in the locality.

In each of the five types of strategy, the concept of 'network' is
central, as a means for understanding the informal ties that it is
sought to tap or to create, and in characterizing the way in which
formal and informal provision can be combined. The term is
central; without it the strategies could not be adequately described
or contrasted with each other. The typology is useful because it
broadens the reference covered by the term, and avoids equating
social support with particular forms of helping such as 'natural
helping networks'.

A different approach to the same set of issues, particularly
salient in North American literature on mental health, is the use of
networks in providing social *support*, with the emphasis upon
support rather than network. A social support network may be
defined as 'a set of interconnected relationships among a group of
people that provides enduring patterns of nurturance in any or all
forms, and provides contingent reinforcement for coping with

life on a day-to-day basis' (Whittaker, 1983, p. 55; see also Pilisuk and Parks, 1986). This is discussed further later in this chapter.

The notion of social network has been pushed to its furthest extreme by American enthusiasts in the social work field who use the term 'networking' to refer to 'a purposeful process of linking three or more people together and of establishing connections and chain reactions among them' (Maguire, 1983, p. 13). It involves professionals working with informal helping networks in the manner described above, except that the process is conceived more actively and in more prescriptive terms.

> People whose relationships or linkages with potentially helpful family and friends are tenuous can be tremendously helped by an informal networker. The social network analyses that allow us to define clearly who should be involved in the helping network, as well as what that person can provide and when it should be provided, are all available. By learning how to analyse a network, help make connections, and support constructive chain reactions, one need not leave to chance what must be done. (Maguire, 1983, p. 23).

Maguire suggests that the active networker starts off with the insights and tools provided by social science to map existing networks and grasp the factual situation, before adding his or her own human judgement or clinical experience to develop a practical strategy which will work in the context of a fluid system of social ties. The technique of personal networking, for example, involves phases of identification, analysis and linking, by which networkers identify potential networks, analyze them and then link the person and the network into a more dense, caring and knowledgeable support system. The networker is the intermediary between the individual and his or her network.

These are some of the more direct applications in the field of community care. Yet an immediate difficulty is apparent: what does the term 'network' actually refer to? Does it not itself become a blanket term, equivalent to saying that all people have some personal ties and close relationships, but tending to tautology? If we are all members of such networks, what is the particular significance of such networks for care? Some of the uses of 'network' just discussed raise serious problems, which will be examined later in this chapter. These difficulties become apparent if one compares these applications to the original uses of this mode of analysis in the social sciences.

SOCIAL NETWORK ANALYSIS

The idea of social network originated in social anthropology. Portraying social relations in terms of a network has a long history, going back at least to A. R. Radcliffe-Brown's definition of social structure as 'a network of actually-existing social relationships' (1940, p. 3). Radcliffe-Brown used the term as a metaphor for the interconnections of social relationships, much as R. M. McIver had earlier talked of the 'web' of social relations. It was a statement that members of society *were* interconnected, without specifying how the nature or form of those links could be used to understand and explain social actions. The beginnings of social network *analysis* lie in the 1950s and early 1960s with the work of John Barnes, Elizabeth Bott and Clyde Mitchell.

Barnes, in his study of a Norwegian island parish (1954) used the concept of social network to denote social relations which were important in the locality but which were not adequately grasped by concepts such as 'community', 'group', or 'occupation'. These relations were primarily ties of friendship and acquaintance which local people partly inherited and partly built up for themselves. Ties with more distant kin, such as cousins, come into the same category.

> Each person is, as it were, in touch with a number of other people, some of whom are directly in touch with each other and some of whom are not. Similarly, each person has a number of friends, and these friends have their own friends; some of any one person's friends know each other, others do not. I find it convenient to talk of a social field of this kind as a *network*. The image I have is of a set of points some of which are joined by lines. The points of the image are people, or sometimes groups, and the lines indicate which people interact with each other. . . . [This is] largely, though not exclusively, a network of ties of kinship, friendship and neighbourhood. This network runs across the whole of society and does not stop at the parish boundary (Barnes, 1954, p. 43).

Elizabeth Bott, in her study of conjugal roles among London families (1957), used social network as a term intermediary between the individual and the family on the one side and the wider society on the other. She suggested the social environments of families were best understood, not as groups of people or the local, geographically-based community, but as networks of relationships. Some might be based on kinship, some on locality, others on occupation. Some friends of a particular family would know each other, others would not. The influence of her study stemmed from the connection she established between her independent variable – whether married couples had 'closed' or 'open' networks – and her dependent variable – segregated or joint conjugal roles.

Although Bott's work stimulated a number of subsequent studies, including hypotheses about the relationship between the character of networks and class imagery (cf. Bulmer, 1975), the setting in which network analysis flourished most successfully was African urban studies. For example, Philip Mayer (1961) contrasted South African black urban migrants who had tight-knit, 'encapsulated' networks which sustained their rural contacts while in towns, and other urban dwellers with more loose-knit networks who also developed closer urban ties while retaining rural links. The former tended to remain rural oriented, the latter became more urban oriented. As developed by Clyde Mitchell in Central Africa, network analysis became a means of coming to terms with the fact that African towns were not single social systems in which all social activities and relationships were necessarily interconnected with each other. It was a means of understanding how the behaviour of people in structured or unstructured situations may be based upon personal ties, the links individuals have with a set of people and the links these people in turn have among themselves and with others (Mitchell, 1966, pp. 54–60).

This development of urban network analysis grew out of a dissatisfaction with the sharp urban-rural contrast postulated in Wirth's 1938 article (discussed in Chapter 2) and a perception that rural migrants in towns did not alter their behaviour so dramatically as to render social patterns in the city totally different from those of the countryside. Network analysis thus grew out of a

dissatisfaction with the analytical frameworks provided by traditional approaches. In sociology, the idea of a simple rural–urban
continuum was decisively rejected. In social anthropology, network analysis was part of a recognition that structural/functional
analysis was inadequate for the understanding of more complex
societies, lacking single pervasive structural characteristics in
terms of which morphologies could be constructed.

Wolfe (1978) has suggested that whereas the main theorists of
Chicago urban sociology, such as Park, Burgess and Wirth,
lacked experience of data gathering through participant observation, the experience of ethnographic fieldwork for African urba-
nists brought home to them the applicability of network analysis.
Certainly this experience conveyed the complexity of urban phenomena and the inadequacy of viewing the town as a single field.
Whether network analysis sprang directly from this ethnographic
experience is more doubtful. As Hannerz (1980) suggests, there
are continuities between Chicago urban sociology and network
analysis, and indeed Elizabeth Bott studied for the Master's
degree in sociology at the University of Chicago in the late 1940s.
John Barnes's background was in mathematics, whence network
analysis has built upon graph theory (cf. Barnes and Harary,
1983). Another tributary was via sociometry and studies of group
dynamics in terms of 'sociograms' (cf. Festinger, Schachter and
Back, 1950). So the emergence of the approach cannot be
attributed primarily to ethnographic experience, though it is true
that in its genesis in the 1950s, social anthropologists played a key
role.

Since the mid-1960s, network analysis has developed rapidly,
with links to a number of disciplines, notably sociology, social
psychology, social anthropology, mathematics and communication theory. The focus here is upon its use in studies of social
support, but it is noteworthy how its potential has been realized in
a variety of different studies, not all of them studies of localities.[1]

A persistent difficulty with network analysis, which particularly afflicts applications in social welfare, is a confusion
between its metaphorical and its analytical use. As a metaphor,
the term was used by Radcliffe-Brown and Warner and Lunt
(1941) talking of a 'network of interrelations . . . of clique
relations' in Yankee City. Meyer Fortes's *Web of Kinship* and R. M.
McIver's web of social relations conveyed a very similar image,

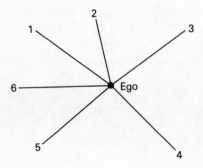

Figure 4.1 Typical Primary Star

without giving the term 'network' any more precise connotation. The step made by Barnes, Bott, Mayer and Mitchell was to use the concept to analyze data and formulate theoretical propositions in terms of the characteristics of the networks of those whom they observed. None of the examples from social welfare cited at the beginning of the chapter do this. 'Network' is used in those examples purely metaphorically, and thus the value and wider applicability of the analyses offered are open to serious question.

The first step to be taken in any proper network *analysis* is to anchor the study to a particular point in the network. Metaphorical use refers to the interconnectedness of the members of society, (in caricature, perhaps, to a 'seamless web'), but for analytical purposes the social scientist must start somewhere and (since the procedures involved become impossibly complex when very large numbers are involved) delimit the parts of the net which are to be studied. This is most usually done by starting from some specified individual whose behaviour or situation the observer wishes to interpret (Mitchell, 1969, pp. 12–15). Bott used networks anchored on two people, the married couple. The person at the centre of the network, on whom it is anchored, is usually designated as 'ego', from whom ties radiate to others.

An important feature of networks is that they are not simply composed of dyadic relations from 'ego' to others. Such a net,

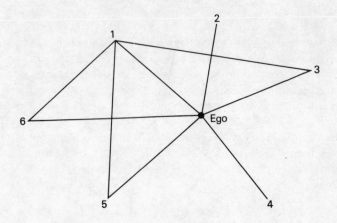

Figure 4.2   Typical Primary Zone

illustrated in Figure 4.1, may be termed a star, and is the starting point for analysis. But a proper network analysis also requires evidence about the direct links between the members of ego's network, independent of ego. These may or may not exist. Figure 4.2 shows a typical network, in which some such links exist and others do not. The aim of network analysis is to focus upon the characteristics of the linkages in the network (rather than the attributes of ego and others) to explain the behaviour of the people involved in them.

Analytically, a network is 'a specific set of linkages among a defined set of persons, with the additional property that the characteristics of these linkages as a whole may be used to interpret the social behaviour of the persons involved' (Mitchell, 1969, p. 2). This requires the collection of data in terms of such networks and their analysis in terms of the form and structure of the networks. This is quite difficult to do, and even well conducted inquiries which appear to make analytical use of the concept may not do so. In Clare Wenger's *The Supportive Network* (1984), for example, a highly regarded study of social support for the elderly in rural North Wales drawn upon in Chapter 3, data are presented on the support network of the dependent elderly. These data are primarily survey responses to questions about persons with whom the respondent is in contact, including separate analyses of contact with children for the elderly who have them. This provides a picture of the contacts which a person has with others (their star), but it does *not* provide a picture of the overall social network within which those individuals are located, particularly of the interconnections between members of the network other than through the person interviewed. How are the other members of this network interconnected? Who are the key persons? Is there any co-ordination among members of the support web? The use of the term 'network' thus remains at a metaphorical level, for the concept implies an attempt to say something about the overall structure of the net not just the links between ego and others in it.

Interactional Features of Networks

So what, analytically, should a network analysis aim to provide? (see Mitchell, 1969; D'Abbs, 1982; Boissevain, 1985). Two types of factor may be identified, structural and interactional, the former referring to the network itself and the latter to its component linkages (Shulman, 1976). The most basic structural factor (about which Wenger *does* provide data) is the *size* of the network. This is made up of two components: direct contacts (sometimes called first-order contacts) and indirect contacts through direct contacts (sometimes called second-order contacts or friends-of-friends – cf. Boissevain, 1974). Most studies focus upon first-order contacts. The size of a network alone, however, is of relatively little interest, and more useful information relates to a variety of interactional features. For each link, information about its *frequency*, *duration* and *durability* is important, though care must be exercised about inferring other consequences from these data. For example, frequency of contact is related to proximity and accessibility, which are important aspects of social support. On the other hand, support may be forthcoming from those with whom ego does not have frequent contact (such as distant kin) while frequent contacts (such as workmates) may not be significant sources of social support. Duration and durability of contacts in a network are distinct from frequency, and may be significant variables in accounting for relationships in a network. For example, contacts among neighbours are greater the longer their length of residence in a particular locality.

In many respects the *content* of a relationship identified within a network is the most important item of information about it. This has several aspects, including the nature of the goods and services exchanged, the closeness or intimacy of the persons linked, the intensity of their interaction, and the exchange of information involved. Boissevain (1974) suggests a concentric zone model of the emotional importance of relationships, whereby respondents are asked to rate subjectively the importance to them of links in their network. At the centre is a personal zone composed of closest relatives and perhaps one or two friends. Each of the other zones signifies decreasing intimacy as one moves outwards. Intensity may be measured in terms of 'closest' ties, or by respondents naming the person to whom they would turn for help in specified situations. Exchanges of goods, services or information need to be elicited to understand the basis of the relationship and what is exchanged, materially or symbolically, between members of the network. Content includes the meanings which people attribute to relationships. These are significant, for 'in the health field they include dimensions of support such as personal or economic assistance; psycho-social activities such as comforting and affirmation of personal importance and role relationships; and the nature of information that is transferred among links' (Chrisman and Kleinman, 1983, p. 578).

Most exchanges in networks are not symmetrical; there is an imbalance of some sort in ties in a network, for example, between husband and wife, or grandparent and grandchild. The *directedness* or *symmetry* of ties needs attention, particularly in studies of social support. It also raises questions about reciprocity which are considered in the next chapter. Asymmetry in transactions between two persons in a network may be an indication of different status (as with grandparents and grandchildren) or differential power (as with spouses) or different interpretations of the nature of the tie (in some contacts between neighbours).

The final important interactional component of ties in a network is the extent to which they display *multiplexity* or *single-strandedness*. Are relations between people single or multiple? This refers to the role(s) played by members of the network and the different capacities in which they interact. If X and Y are in contact, do they know one another simply as (1) neighbours or (2) fellow-members of a voluntary association or (3) workmates or (4) friends? Studies of rural villages and of traditional urban working-class communities have demonstrated very high degrees of multiplexity, particularly in enclosed rural or mining communities. In common-sense terms it is often said that 'everyone knows everyone else'. What this means analytically is that there is overlap between kinship, being neighbours, working together, spending leisure time together, worshipping together, belonging to the same associations, and in the past having grown up together and gone to the same school. Such complete overlapping of ties is nowadays highly unusual, and indeed the Simmel-Wirth view of urban life postulated the breakdown of such multiplex ties into single-stranded relations, where those who were interacted with in one setting (for example, work) were not interacted with in other contexts. Such atomism in urban life lies at the opposite end of the continuum to the multiplex ties of the enclosed agricultural or mining community. The interesting empirical question is where, between these two extremes, do modern urban dwellers lie? As already noted, a good deal of doubt has been thrown on the Wirthian view of atomism. The precise extent of continuing multiplexity in relationships is a subject requiring empirical inquiry in particular cases, the results of which are relevant to the availability of social support.

Structural Features of Networks

Turning to structural features of a network other than size, the most important is *density*. This refers to the extent to which members of a person's network are in touch with each other independently of ego. It is the feature of networks that has been most often highlighted, usually in terms of a contrast between tight-knit and loose-knit networks, or networks of small and large mesh. Density can be expressed in formal terms as the proportion of links which actually exist in a network compared to the links which could possibly exist. This measure is a measure of the links connecting all persons in a network with each other, not simply of the ties between ego and the other members of his network. Empirically, gathering data of this sort is a very formidable undertaking, the number of ties increasing exponentially as the size of the network increases. For example, between four people there are a maximum of six ties possible (treating each line joining two people as one tie), whereas with 20 people, there are 171 possible ties among the 20, *excluding* ego's own relationship to the 19 others.

Density has usually been considered to be a significant sociological variable. Generally, the assumption has been that the higher the density of a network, the greater the social communication among its members, resulting both in greater social support (there is more extensive knowledge of the needs of members of the network) and greater social control (any form of deviance is more widely known and subject to informal social pressures). Bott's study suggested that density was the significant independent variable explaining variation in conjugal roles. A study by Wellman in Toronto, however, showed that in his data density was not related to the availability of social support. According to this view,

> primary ties are often dispersed among multiple, sparsely inter-connected social networks . . . primary ties now tend to form sparsely-knit, spatially dispersed, ramifying structures instead of being bound up within a single densely-knit solidarity. While such ties may have fewer strands in the relationship than those in which kinship, residence and work are combined, they are prevalent and important sources of sociability and support (Wellman, 1979, p. 1207).

A recent study of friendship and social support in a London suburb (Willmott, 1987) also suggests that high density of networks is not necessarily associated with higher levels of support. A further point of note is that when more extended networks are being examined, there is likely to be variation in density across the network. Some parts may be more dense than others.

Two other structural features of networks may also lead to variation across the network. *Clustering* is the degree to which some members of a network form clusters of persons who are more closely linked to one another than they are to the rest of the network. *Reachability* refers to the accessibility of others in the network by the number of steps between ego and specified others in the network. If the proportion of people who can be contacted in a small number of steps is large, then the network is more compact compared to one in which a larger number of steps are needed.

The point of this rather extended discussion of the structural and interactional characteristics of networks is to emphasize the difference between metaphorical and analytic uses of the term 'social network'. If one seeks to use the term analytically, then the various characteristics of networks need to be investigated to make sense of the patterns one discovers. This is a complex methodological task (cf. Mitchell, 1969, pp. 30–36; D'Abbs, 1982, Part 2) but before embarking upon it one needs to be clear what it is one is investigating. Such understanding tends to be clouded or entirely obscured in the purely metaphorical use of the term 'network' in the community care literature.

SOCIAL SUPPORT

A further aspect to be considered is the discussion of the role of networks in the provision of social support. Social support and social networks have increasingly been linked in recent discussions of how social care can be provided outside institutions.

> Support is furnished by a helper (who may or may not be a professional) who is accepted as an ally by the distressed individual. It consists of the communication, sometimes non-verbal, by the helper that the helper's training, experience and understanding are at the service of the distressed individual as the latter struggles to regain equilibrium (Weiss, 1976, p. 215).

Robert Weiss has further elaborated the approach in terms of components of support (1969; 1975), which is discussed at the beginning of the next chapter.

The study of the impact of social support upon the state of distressed or dependent individuals has been pursued furthest in research into physical and mental health. Two particularly influential researchers have been John Cassel, an epidemiologist, and Gerald Caplan, a specialist in community health. Cassel hypothesized (1974) that there was a social feedback mechanism from people's social environment to people's resistance to disease. Certain kinds of change in social environment could trigger metabolic effects, increasing vulnerability, while health could be protected by certain social supports provided by the primary groups of most importance to the individual. Caplan identified the importance of relationship durability as one hallmark of a system of supportive ties, made up of significant others.

> The significant others help the individual mobilize his psychological resources and master his emotional burdens; they share his tasks; and they supply him with extra supplies of money, materials, tools, skills, and cognitive guidance to improve his handling of his situation. (Caplan 1974, p. 6)

Such social supports can act as a buffer against the onset of disease. When populations are studied, statistically significant variations may appear related to such support.

A number of studies have demonstrated the existence of a relationship between support and lower incidence of pathology (cf. Pilisuk and Parks, 1986). Berkman and Syme (1979), for example, in a well-known paper showed in a nine-year follow up of residents of Almeda County, California, that there was a marked association between social ties and mortality. People who lacked social and community ties were considerably more likely to die in the follow-up period than those with more extensive contacts. Other studies have reported that social support contributes to buffering stress, and therefore to reducing illness, though the precise mechanisms by which this occurs are unclear. Such studies include Gore's (1978) study of the health consequences of unemployment, Nuckolls *et al.*'s (1982) study of complications in pregnancy among army wives, and Brown and Harris's (1978) study of depression among working-class married women.

Though the association between support and outcome is established for many pathological conditions, the precise causal factors operating are obscure. One commentary distinguishes between 'social interaction', 'social support', and 'stress', and suggests that the three are not infrequently confounded. 'Some changes in life circumstances that are treated as "stressful events" also represent changes in social interaction and social support. For example, death of a spouse and divorce are stressful events, but they also represent changes in a person's pattern of social interaction, and social support' (Specht, 1986, p. 223). Moreover, it can be argued that the causal relationship might run in the other direction, from health to wider social ties. People may be more likely to interact with, and support, people who are happy and competent and these happier and more competent people are less likely to experience stress. Links between social support and health are thus in need of much further research, and there is a good deal of uncertainty about precisely how social relationships influence health outcome (cf. Thoits, 1982; Ell, 1984).

To the study of social support has been added more recently approaches in terms of social networks, as a complementary means of understanding the way in which social behaviour might influence health. An influential early study, by McKinlay (1973), showed how variation in types of network could influence patterns of utilization of health services. 'Social network' is more specific than 'social support', referring to a specific set of interrelated persons. Moreover, network analysis emphasizes

> 'the asymmetric, multi-faceted nature of ties and the importance of structural patterns. By treating the content of these ties as flows of resources, it transforms the study of support into supportive resources, and it links the allocation of these resources to large-scale social phenomena' (Wellman, 1981, p. 179).

Thus it can take account of asymmetry and reciprocity in ties within a network more precisely than can a conceptualization in terms of social support. It also avoids interpreting behaviour solely on the basis of relationships between two people – dyads – since it takes account of the larger web of which they are part.

In some work of this type, 'network' has been used in a purely metaphorical way, with little consequent gain in understanding. In other studies, however, it has been used in a more precise analytical sense. McKinlay's study of health seeking behaviour (1973) is one instance. A review of research on schizophrenia by Hammer (1981) suggested that the social networks of schizophrenic individuals tend to be smaller than those of normal individuals, and non-kin in those networks are internally less interconnected than in normal networks, seeming to have fewer connections with kin clusters. Schizophrenic individuals also had more asymmetric and fewer multiplex relationships than non-psychotic controls. Gottleib (1981) has demonstrated how network analysis can be used in the study of mental illness. And Wellman has used his East York data, and other sources, to suggest that support is more complex than is sometimes supposed (Wellman, 1981; Wellman and Hiscott, 1985). In particular, the assumption that densely knit networks are necessarily related to access to more support and better health is not proven, while social ties can perform multiple functions, both positive and negative, with varying implications for health (Hall and Wellman, 1985). For example, participation in a peer group culture which engages in heavy smoking and drinking in the course of convivial sociability will make it more difficult for individuals within the group to alter their behaviour. They are subject to network support of a negative kind, and such social and cultural influences upon health behaviour are of considerable significance.

THE USE OF NETWORK ANALYSIS TO STUDY CARE AND SUPPORT

How have studies of social networks been applied to the study of informal care and support systems? Four examples will be considered in which analytic use is made of the concept of network to understand ways in which social support is provided.

Carol Stack's anthropological study, *All Our Kin* (1974), addressed the question of how female-headed black families coped with life in an inner-city housing estate in a mid-western American city. Many previous studies, by E. F. Frazier (1939), St Clair Drake and Horace Cayton (1945) and Rainwater (1966), as well as the controversial Moynihan Report of 1965 (Rainwater and Yancey, 1967), had emphasized that illegitimacy and female-headed households were symptomatic of broken homes and family disorganization. Stack showed that while ties with spouses and relatives might be weak, poor black families evolved quasi-kin relations with fellow residents, with whom they formed kinship-based exchange networks linking multiple domestic units. Seen in this light, the fatherless black family was not a case of social disorganization and social pathology but of tenacious adaptation to economic adversity and lower class position. Stack was able to demonstrate these connections through intensive analysis of the networks linking different families within a particular locality.

She emphasized particularly the importance of the exchanges

between poor families whose own resources were generally meagre and derived from the welfare system.

Black families living in The Flats (the locale of the study) need a steady source of cooperative support to survive. They share with one another because of the urgency of their needs. Alliances between individuals are created around the clock as kin and friends exchange and give and obligate one another. They trade food stamps, rent money, a TV, hats, dice, a car, a nickel here, a cigarette there, food, milk, grits and children. . . . The resources, possessions and services exchanged between individuals residing in The Flats are intricately interwoven. People exchange various objects generously: new things, treasured items, furniture, cars, goods that are perishable, and services that are exchanged for child care, residence, or shared meals. Individuals enlarge their web of social relations through repetitive and seemingly habitual instances of swapping. . . . Through exchange transactions, an individual personally mobilises others as participants in his social network (Stack, 1974, pp. 32, 33–4, 43).

Some of these exchanges took place with other relatives living in the same area, others with close friends who had come to be granted the status of quasi-kin. It is the use of these personal ties as a means of mobilizing social support which underlies the criticism of theories of the pathological or socially disorganized black family. Reciprocal gift-giving joins individuals in personal relationships, most adequately represented as a network. A network perspective is then used to interpret the interpersonal links among those individuals who exchange goods and services to solve daily domestic problems.

Reciprocity is at the heart of the process. Individuals who do not reciprocate are judged harshly. Stack describes the continual flow of goods and services back and forth between people in a network, often on a daily, or even hourly, basis. Everyone is well informed about the financial circumstances of others in their network and there is an expectation that what comes in will be shared. This style of gift exchange, based on interpersonal relationships rooted in local coalitions of co-operating kin and quasi-kin, is in contrast to that of working-class blacks in employment or to the middle-class ethic of individualism. No one in the network is turned down when they need help, and in the long run everyone comes out about equal. In the short term, however, network exchanges are a means of keeping adversity at bay and, argues Stack, a profoundly creative adaptation to poverty. The co-operative life style and the bonds created by the vast mass of day-to-day exchanges constitute an underlying element in black identity.

Stack's study is in the mould of Elizabeth Bott's study, in the sense of being a detailed analysis of a small number of cases with little attempt to measure quantitatively. Nevertheless it provides rich data upon the frequency, duration, direction and symmetry of network ties, and particularly upon their content. Stack demonstrates what support involves and the exchanges involved for those who participate. Particularly relevant to the field of care is the way in which adult females on the estate co-operate in the care of children, not just in looking after each other's children but sometimes in having children go to live temporarily in other families at times of domestic difficulty. Here, the significance of friends who become quasi-kin (treated as if they were kin) becomes apparent, for they are integrated into the kin-structured domestic networks through which support in the care of children is provided. Stack's study is far from unique as a study of black family life in the ghetto (for a contrasting study see Susser, 1982; and for a general review Malson, 1982), but it is unusual in the fruitful way in which it uses network analysis both as a method and as an explanatory factor in examining its subject.

The second example may be considered more briefly. It bears on the discussion of loneliness in the previous chapter. Neena Chappell (1983) studied informal support networks among the elderly in Winnipeg, Canada. The data are derived from a random sample of 400 elderly individuals in the city, interviewed at home, stratified by age and sex to ensure a sufficient number of elderly men in the sample. Four-fifths had lived in Winnipeg for twenty years or more. Although 15 per cent of the sample reported having no close friends, and 16 per cent only one, the majority had a considerable number, most of whom were elderly themselves, that is, age peers. The significant finding in terms of social ties was that contact with close friends was more common than with relatives living outside the household. Two-thirds of the sample saw their friends at least once a month. High levels of satisfaction with these friendships were expressed.

Linked to data on family contacts, the study emphasized the importance of social ties among peers (that is, those of the same age).

> Friends tend to be age peers. That is, the importance of peers (family peers within the household and non-family as friends) among those available in these elderly persons' social network is clear (Chappell, 1983, pp. 95–6).

This has considerable implications for social care, and is consistent with evidence that a large proportion of informal carers of the elderly are themselves elderly. Chappell's study does not provide extensive data on networks, but provides some suggestive initial findings as pointers to further research.

The third example is Marc Granovetter's now classic paper, 'The strength of weak ties' (1973). He defined the strength of a tie as the combination of the amount of time, the emotional intensity, the intimacy, mutual confiding and the reciprocal services which characterize the tie. Strong ties are those which are embedded in dense social networks in which a high proportion of the members are in contact with each other independently. He points out that dense networks tie people into tightly knit sets of relationships that limit their contacts with people who have information and knowledge about how to function in social contexts removed from their primary relationships. 'Weak' ties are ties which bridge between primary networks which may or may not themselves be 'strong'. They are typically ties from an individual (ego) to others who are not tied to others in ego's network, but are tied into networks of their own, to which ego can gain access through them. Granovetter demonstrates this process at work through the process of job search, which showed that those to whom job searchers were weakly tied were more help in finding jobs because they moved in other circles and had access to information different from that held by the people in contact with them. The results are also generalized to a macro-level:

> Social systems lacking in weak ties will be fragmented and incoherent. New ideas will spread slowly, scientific endeavours will be handicapped, and subgroups that are separated by

race, ethnicity, geography and other characteristics will have difficulty reaching a modus vivendi (Granovetter, 1983, p. 202).

An early version of the original paper was entitled 'Alienation reconsidered', and the argument runs counter to the Wirthian view of the consequences of modern urbanism. Far from the urban isolate becoming *déracinée* (separated from one's roots), such loose-knit and far-flung networks could be functional for effective social participation. Two studies in the area of social support lend further support to this view. Wilcox (1981) found that divorced women were more likely to make successful social or emotional adjustments if their pre-divorce social networks were less dense than divorced women who had dense pre-divorce networks. B. J. Hirsch (1981) similarly found greater flexibility in studies of young widows and women returning to study after being housewives. Loose-knit networks seemed to give people in those situations more room to manoeuvre, and were less constraining than if they remained within a fairly narrow circle in which their role was a limited one (so and so's ex-wife, for example).

It may thus be hypothesized, contrary to Wirth, that weak ties are indispensable to individuals' opportunities and to their integration into communities. Strong ties, breeding local cohesion, lead to overall fragmentation. Weak ties do not generate alienation. If this is so, it has particular relevance for the study of neighbourly relations, which typically tend to be weaker than those with kin. Whether ties of friendship are stronger or weaker than kin ties depends on sex, age and social class. Ties with neighbours are not, in any case, generally the most important personal relationships in an individual's network. Yet for some forms of support in the community – for example, enabling the infirm elderly to remain living at home – such weak ties with neighbours may be of considerable importance in providing individuals with particular forms of care. Interesting propositions derived from this may be tested, such as that the intensity of neighbourly relations varies directly with the intensity of kin relations, and not inversely. Those with stronger kinship networks would also have stronger neighbouring relations, while those with weaker kinship networks would also tend to be more isolated from their neighbours.

In more recent reflections upon the theory, however, Granovetter has entered a caveat so far as lower class and lower income groups are concerned. He was struck by parallels between Stack's study and a study by Larissa Lomnitz of a shanty town on the edge of Mexico City (1977), which found reciprocity between neighbours bound together in a kinship network as the basis of economic survival. Poor people clearly rely on strong ties more than others do. A study in Philadelphia by Ericksen and Yancey (1977) concludes that those who maintain stronger networks tend to be younger, less well-educated, and black.

> This pervasive use of strong ties by the poor and insecure is a response to economic pressures; they believe themselves to be without alternatives, and the adaptive nature of these reciprocity networks is the main theme of the analysts. At the same time . . . the heavy concentration of social energy in strong ties has the effect of fragmenting communities of the poor into encapsulated networks with poor connections between these units; individuals so encapsulated may then lose some of the advantages associated with the outreach of weak ties. This may be one more reason why poverty is self-perpetuating (Granovetter, 1983, p. 213).

The fourth example of the use of network analysis is by Bruce Kapferer, the Manchester social anthropologist, in his study of Zambian industrial workers (1969, 1972). Critics of network analysis have charged that although many fascinating new ways of describing interaction have been produced, there has been little progress with the main project of explaining content in terms of form. Many of the findings of network studies which claim to show relationships between the formal properties of networks and behaviour are highly tentative or contested, or both. Philip Abrams, for example, observed that:

> one of the main reasons why so many of the proposed relationships between density and other factors cannot be found effectively in the real world is, . . . as Kapferer (and others) have argued, precisely because density . . . has to be measured in terms of *all* the links in a network. The varying content of

actual links is deliberately ignored; equal weight is given to all links, regardless of the varying significance they might have for all concerned. If one recognises that different links can have widely different values for individuals within a network, one may get much closer to an explanation of the relationships in which one is interested but the explanation is no longer grounded in the notion of density as a formal property of interaction; it is an explanation of the significant content of relationships, not of the structure of networks (Bulmer, 1986a, p. 89).

Thus, applied to Bott's study, it may be argued that density itself may not be an adequate independent variable, and has to be explained in turn in terms of occupation, social and geographical mobility, ethnic origin, education and family life cycle phase. Lockwood's work on class imagery (1966) and the research stemming from it (Bulmer, 1975) exemplifies such an enlargement of focus.

Kapferer's work takes on an added significance in the light of this critique. He sought to develop explanations of the closeness or connectedness of members of networks in terms of the significance or value of their interactions, and in addition to draw attention to the *exchange* element in relationships in trying to account for their significance. Like Michael Anderson's study of nineteenth-century Preston (1971), his work represented an attempt to specify the content of relationships in terms of the exchange of services and the mutual advantage that each party derived from the exchange. It also connects in a very interesting way with what may be called the sociology of altruism – for example, in Alvin Gouldner's formulation (1973) of the norm of beneficence. To what extent are relations between workmates, neighbours, kin or friends conditioned by the give and take involved? This is a broad issue but network analysis provides an appropriate framework for its elucidation when studying informal social care. Kapferer's study underlines the need in studies of social support to focus on the resources exchanged in the network, and the exchanges, costs and rules which operate within it. Form alone – in particular, exclusive concentration upon structural characteristics such as size and density – cannot satisfactorily explain variations in social support.

NETWORK ANALYSIS ASSESSED

These four studies, then, demonstrate the potential for properly conducted network analyses to illuminate social processes and throw light on the provisions of community care. It cannot be gainsayed, however, that the promise of network analysis has so far exceeded what it has delivered, and a critical assessment of the approach, both from the point of view of its proponents and of those who would apply it to the study of social support, is now in order.

Network analysis can clearly mean rather different things. There is a marked difference between small-scale, qualitative suggestive studies such as those of Bott (1957) and Stack (1974), more quantitative studies such as those of Laumann (1973) and Fischer (1982), and technical formalizations of network analysis, drawing on graph and balance theories, whose aim is primarily methodological (see, for example, many of the articles in the journal *Social Networks*).

Bridging the gap between method and substance can be particularly difficult. Indeed, one major criticism is that network analysis emphasizes form at the expense of content. A map of the ties connecting one individual to others in their network, or of the ties connecting members of a particular collectivity, is of little use unless one also knows what the content of those ties is. Perhaps this is one reason why certain qualitative network studies have had great impact, because in such intensive studies it is easier to combine analysis of content with that of form. Methods of analyzing content are being developed. The promise is there, and particularly for more applied work network analysis could make a considerable contribution. It has great potential for explaining the organization of sociability and support, yet surprisingly this potential remains unfulfilled (Allan, 1979, p. 126).

One reason is undoubtedly that collecting sufficient data about networks, particularly where these exceed a few people, is very time-consuming and in some cases beyond the efforts of a single investigator. Another is that the technique may rather too easily become an end in itself, rather than a means to answering substantive social science questions. One anthropological network analyst, Jeremy Boissevain, is scathing about the over-elaboration of technique and data, and the use of a battery of techniques which results in overkill. 'Flies are killed with dynamite' (Boissevain, 1979, p. 393). His critique of the use of jargon, theory and techniques borrowed from mathematical graph theory has been strongly contested (Barnes and Harary, 1983), but such differences among network analysts are indicative of the problems of methodological complexity.

There is a sense, too, in which, particularly from the formalistic studies, so much is promised and so little delivered. Some have argued that it leads to triviality. 'Networks are compared with regard to density, size, and even composition, much in the way butterfly-collectors compare the colouring, wingspread and number of spots of their favourite species' (Boissevain, 1979, p. 393). Boissevain's ire seems to be directed particularly at sociologists, but the possibility of special pleading should not detract from the force of the criticism. Mapping networks in themselves does not amount to much unless linked to particular scientific problems. Networks need to be studied for a purpose, not just for their form. To show, for example, network links between overlapping directorships, or between politicians and *mafiosi* does not necessarily demonstrate collusion, without data on the actual exchanges that take place within those networks. Similarly, to map the informal network of an individual and his or her ties with kin, friends and neighbours does not tell one very much about the types of aid and support which might be provided to that individual in adversity.

A more general claim made by some network analysts is that the approach constitutes a new way of understanding the structural properties which affect behaviour. They claim that it constitutes a new theoretical approach.

> Network analysts . . . concentrate on studying how the pattern of ties in a network provides significant opportunities and constraints because it affects the access of people and institutions to such resources as information, wealth and power. Thus network analysts treat social systems as networks of dependency relationships resulting from the differential possession of scarce resources at the nodes and the structural allocation of these resources at the ties (Wellman, 1983, p. 157).

This claim to have developed a new form of structural analysis is not particularly convincing, at least as yet. 'There is no "network theory" in the sense of a set of logically interrelated, testable propositions' (Hannerz, 1980, p. 175).

How successfully has network analysis been applied to policy issues? Here several issues have to be faced rather sharply. At least its pure academic practitioners have used the concept precisely and analytically, whereas practitioners in the applied field, as the opening examples in this chapter have suggested, have used it much more broadly. A severe critic might even claim that 'network' has been all things to all men, and so devoid of meaning that 'tie' or 'relationship' could be substituted for it. This is too severe, but a more substantial criticism is that its use in applied settings has remained to a large extent metaphorical rather than analytical. This metaphorical usage is widespread. A perceptive discussion of community care policy by Olive Stevenson, for example, refers to 'the need to know more about the social networks upon which the development of community care must rest' (Stevenson, 1980, p. 27) but says no more about what those networks are or how they might be used. A thoughtful survey of 'community networks' by Jack Rothman and Donald Warren (1981), although referring to some of the network literature, uses the term 'network' largely as a metaphor, and shades off into discussion of 'natural support systems', a dubious concept. A recent symposium with the title *Support Networks in a Caring Community* (Yoder, Jonker and Leaper, 1985) confines itself, with the exception of one paper by Benjamin Gottleib, either to the purely metaphorical use of 'network' or to no use at all. It is as if the term is used to label the problem or area to be discussed but is not then followed through to exploit its analytic potential.

The possibility has to be faced that 'network' is in danger of becoming simply a synonym for 'community', reintroducing that difficult term in a different guise. The Barclay Report of 1982 comes close to doing this, for it identifies community with local networks of formal and informal relationships. The straitjacket it puts itself into is by assuming that such networks are *local*. This cuts away one of the great virtues of the network approach, 'its sensitivity to the particularity of context. It leaves open the question of whether a specific social aggregate is a community or not. It is an empirical question to determine whether a neighbourhood is a community or not' (Bender, 1978, p. 123). Barclay does not treat this as an empirical question (Allan, 1983, pp. 420–1). It would be much more fruitful if applied network researchers could apply some of the insights of urban sociology, which has used network analysis to search for linkages and flow of resources, *before* tying them to particular spatial patterns. Wellman and Leighton's useful contrast (1979) between theories of community 'lost', community 'saved' and community 'liberated', for example, (see pp. 103–6) would have given the Barclay Committee some real purchase on underlying social trends, instead of using a formulation in terms of informal social networks (that is, local community ties) which is either circular or more or less vacuous.

Another trap which some applied researchers fall into is to hypothesize networks as real entities, into which voluntary or statutory services may be 'plugged' or which may be 'tapped' as the need arises. Maguire's book (1983) quoted earlier tends in this direction, with its facile appeal to 'networking'. Such uses of the network idea are simplistic and misleading. Price's caution is worth attending to:

> Esoteric network analysis can be profoundly misleading when transposed into applied research agendas without specification of the assumptions on which such work is founded. [Some] policy makers and welfare agents . . . apparently proceed as if there were ready formulae for the practical application of the idea of a social network to facilitate social intervention. Despite a contrary impression in some quarters, it is not constructive to regard the networks of empirical research as objectively real, in the sense that they are available 'to tap into' or for that matter to be readily replicated (Price, 1981, pp. 304–5).

Nor, feminists would add, are helping networks 'natural'.

The delicacy and fragility of informal networks in society needs to be emphasized. This is most apparent between neighbours. Neighbours relate to each other by virtue of the fact of co-residence. If a neighbour moves away, contact is lost unless the relationship had previously been transformed into one of friendship. There is good evidence that one of the most important factors fostering ties between neighbours is length of residence. The longer they have lived near each other, the more likelihood of contact once they move away. A formal organization such as the DHSS is in a difficult position trying to 'tap' such a tie, or 'plug in' to it, indeed when dealing with dependent clients there is probably a greater chance that such intervention may disrupt the tie than build upon it. Coward (1982) has cautioned against too rapid or optimistic intervention in relation to informal networks supporting the dependent elderly. Some of the issues of how to 'interweave' formal and informal care are pursued in Chapter 6.

The Barclay Report made no attempt to consider the organization and content of different types of informal relationship, but treated all informal ties as on a par with each other. Despite considerable research on the subject, the Report treats any relationship in which an individual is involved as having a potential for becoming incorporated into a system of informal caring. Research into kinship, friendship and neighbouring ties suggests that this is most unlikely. For example, neighbour relations are not particularly well suited to the Barclay model of drawing on informal networks.

> Consistent caring (between one neighbour and another) is not an extension of neighbour relations but a break from their routine patterning. It would create a greater dependence, a reduction in privacy, and of course the possibility of public recognition of one's private troubles. . . . More personal forms of caring become problematic because they involve a degree of intrusion into personal life that lies well outside the normal rules of neighbouring. To the extent that aid is given, it cannot occur between people who are *just* neighbours as the neighbour bond is normally defined in far too limited a fashion (Allan, 1983, p. 429).

Most applied discussions of informal networks also ignore the political and economic dimensions of informal support. Here the work of Philip Abrams on neighbours (Bulmer, 1986a) is particularly pertinent, for he sought to tie the discussion of neighbourhood care to the question of local community organization. Indeed, his concept of modern neighbourhoodism explicitly included local political organization. Moreover, network analysis may be used to illuminate the structure of local decision making (cf. Laumann and Pappi, 1976) and expose the sociological realities underlying political manifestations. One interesting hypothesis to examine concerning the strength of weak ties is as follows. The more local bridges there are (that is, weak ties) between different social networks in a neighbourhood, the more cohesive it is likely to be and the more capable of acting in concert.

Those seeking to apply network analysis need to remember that:

> supportive networks do not operate in a vacuum, nor is the infusion of resources for social support a matter that can be adequately addressed simply at the local level. Self-help is neither selfless nor cheap. Family and community effectiveness in the provision of social support is heavily dependent upon the broader economic and social environment. . . . Indeed, to overemphasize the singular influence of social ties on health and well-being, and to ignore the broader context within which those social ties operate, constitutes a political misuse of the findings on the social support and health relationship (Pilisuk and Minkler, 1985, p. 11).

It is not sufficient, then, for the Barclay Report simply to invoke 'social networks' as the key to unlocking the mysteries of community care. Social network analysis is a way of understanding the patterning of social ties which pertain neither to a group nor to an institution. In the social care field social network analysis has – with one or two exceptions such as Carol Stack – been used in a loose metaphorical sense which has added little to our understanding of the capacity of care to be provided on the basis of personal ties. Charles Froland's distinctions between different strategies using networks (see pp. 113–14) is useful, but does not describe how such networks are to be identified, still less linked into.

What is needed now are attempts to use analytic network methods to study empirically social support and social care. Several such works in the health field have been cited, but there are fewer studies in the personal social services. They are urgently needed, for social network analysis does have considerable potential, provided that it is remembered that it is essentially a sophisticated mapping technique. Barclay's vision of social workers becoming 'upholders of networks' may be doubted for some of the reasons suggested in this and the previous chapter. Knowing more about such social ties around an individual – both local and non-local – is an essential prerequisite to planning integrated care, and this is a theme which is taken up in Chapter 6.

NOTES

1 These include Bruce Kapferer's study of a Zambian factory (1972), Edward Laumann and E. O. Pappi's monograph on a German town (1976), Marc Granovetter's study of job searching (1974), John McKinlay's analysis of channels of seeking health care (1973), Carol Stack's ethnography of the black extended family in America (1974) and Claude Fischer's *To Dwell Among Friends* (1982), which is the closest to mainstream urban sociology. All these studies show the value of studying networks independently of either structural concepts such as 'group' or geographically-based entities such as 'community'. The approach has been used most intensively, perhaps, by anthropologists and sociologists associated with Max Gluckman and the Rhodes-Livingstone Institute: Barnes, Mitchell, David Boswell, Peter Harries-Jones, Kapferer and others, using the metaphors of close knit–loose knit, or multiplex–single stranded. Except in Mitchell's work, this approach was not highly formalized, rather, it was suggestive of ways in which people's informal social relationships modified under conditions of social change.

5

The Philosophical and Sociological Bases of Caring

The discussion so far has concentrated upon social structural aspects of informal social care. What of the motives and values of carers? Why do they provide personal care of various kinds? What is the basis of the personal ties which bind people to each other and lead to caring? These are broad questions, of a philosophical as well as sociological and psychological nature, which need to be tackled even if no definitive answers are possible. For the attempt to answer them may provide some clues as to *why* carers care, which is very necessary to understand if policies in this area are to be soundly based.

> Alongside the increasing longevity which most of us welcome has come a phenomenon unknown in previous centuries, which is therefore something that the human race simply hasn't learned to live with. The art of living with chronic illness and disability is something we have few patterns for. . . . We have to invent new ways to live with long-term stress, caused by the unpredictability and unpleasant manifestations of these conditions (Briggs and Oliver, 1985, pp. xv–xvi).

Caring, after all, is work, and often arduous work. Physical tending, in particular, can be very strenuous, and can place a considerable burden upon the carer. Some types of dependency – senile dementia in the elderly, extreme physical disability, certain kinds of mental handicap – may require more or less continuous attendance and may not permit the person cared for to be left for any significant length of time. This places great strains upon the carer (cf. EOC, 1982), yet people provide such care for those to whom they are linked by personal ties despite the costs to themselves.

THE PROVISIONS OF SOCIAL RELATIONSHIPS

Why do individuals maintain personal relationships with others? This question is at the heart of the caring process, and needs to be explored thoroughly if that process is to be properly understood. Generalized explanations such as 'because she's my mother', 'because he needs me', or 'no one else could manage her', need probing to find out why people provide the care they do. Robert Weiss has outlined and tested two alternative theories of caring: the idea of a 'fund of sociability' and the notion of a 'mediating primary group'. The fund of sociability concept holds that individuals have a readiness and need to interact with others. The need may be distributed in various ways but is a constant amount (cf. Nelson, 1966; Bott, 1957). Individuals may, with equal satisfaction, engage in a great deal of intense contact with a few people or more limited less intense contact with a great many others. The theory of mediating primary groups, on the other hand, draws on the distinction between close, frequent, face-to-face and emotionally loaded ties which are primary, and instrumental, affectively neutral ties which are secondary (as in the world of work). This theory holds that people's beliefs, attitudes and understandings were formed in primary groups to which they once belonged – for example, in their family of origin, and among peers in adolescence and early adulthood – and are now maintained through interaction with others in other primary groups to which these people now belong.

Weiss's research on lone parents suggested that neither theory was adequate. There was no support for the fund of sociability idea, for relationships were differentiated and one type was not an adequate substitute for another. 'In the absence of membership in a social network which shared their central life concerns, individuals experience severe distress' (Weiss, 1975, p. 21). The provisions of marriage could not be supplied by friendship. (As one respondent put it: 'Sometimes I have the girls over and we talk about how hard it is, Misery loves company.') Nor could the provisions of friendship be supplied by marriage. But for the same reason, the primary-secondary distinction proved inadequate. Marriage and friendship are both close, face-to-face, primary relationships, yet what they provide is distinct and the two are not alternatives. As Litwak and Szelenyi argued (1969), different primary group ties perform different functions.

Weiss was led to conclude that individuals have requirements for well-being that can be met only through relationships. Individuals maintain relationships to gain provisions. But different relational provisions depend upon different, and usually incompatible, relational assumptions. Thus, a relationship with a friend, a child and a spouse all rest on different bases, and a degree of specialization occurs in what is provided by a particular relationship. Unlike the discussion earlier of the role of kin, friends and neighbours, Weiss's typology (1969, 1975) addresses the emotional and cognitive needs to be met rather than the social roles played. The six types are as follows.

1   *Attachment and intimacy* is provided in relationships from which individuals gain a sense of security and place. Feelings can be expressed freely and without self-consciousness, and in such relationships individuals feel comfortable and at home. The absence of such relationships is likely to lead to loneliness and restlessness. Attachment is provided by marriage or other sustained sexual partnership, in some close relationships between a woman and a close friend, sister or mother; and for some men in relationships with 'buddies'.

2   *Social integration* is provided by relationships in which participants share concerns because they are in the same situation or striving for similar objectives, and can exchange experience, information and ideas. This may be provided by friends or work colleagues. In the area of social support, self-help groups may often provide a means for the social integration of the otherwise isolated person.

3 Opportunities for *nurturance,* where an adult takes responsibility for a child, encourages the development of a sense of being needed, and may also provide a model for care in the future (for example, by a daughter or son of an elderly parent).

4 *Reassurance of worth* is provided by relationships that demonstrate an individual's competence in some role. This may be provided by work, or for men by the ability to support and defend a family. The loss of a source of such reassurance is likely to result in decreased self-esteem, as, for example, for unemployed heads of families.

5 *Reliable assistance* through the provision of services or resources being made available. Friends and/or neighbours may be a source at some period and in some circumstances, but it is only among close kin that continued assistance may be expected regardless of the affective ties. This pattern is particularly evident in patterns of informal support for the elderly. Absence of a relationship offering such assistance is likely to be reflected in increased anxiety and vulnerability.

6 *Obtaining guidance* is derived from relationships with respected others, such as priests, doctors, nurses, social workers and counsellors (cf. Weiss, 1973b), and on occasion impersonal advice services which do not involve face-to-face contact.

Weiss argues that the relationship that provides attachment is of central importance in the organization of one's life. Individuals will tend to organize their life around those relationships which provide them with attachment – usually with a spouse or partner, but it could be a grown child or a close friend. Other relationships are then integrated with this central relationship. Lack of an intimate relationship may have distressing consequences, as Brown and Harris (1978) have shown in linking the absence of such ties with the development of depression among working-class women.

From the point of view of care, several of these types of relationship play a significant part. Particularly among the dependent elderly, relationships of attachment provide the basis for sustained care, not just between spouses but between close friends or relatives (such as siblings) who have kept house together for a long period. When such a relationship ends with the death of one party, emotional isolation and desolation often results, even if other social relationships are maintained. Reliable assistance is very important in enabling many types of dependent person to continue living in the community, and parts of the preceding discussion have been concerned with the extent to which kin, neighbours and friends may be expected to provide such support. Social integration may be particularly important for some – for example, families with young children, and families with a mentally handicapped member – and its absence can lead to social isolation and loneliness. The experience of being nurtured has received insufficient attention in discussions of care, and will be returned to below. The value of Weiss's approach lies in asking what emotional and relational provisions different relationships offer, opening up a discussion of different values underlying caring and grounding the discussion in actual patterns of social relationships.

One useful way forward is to relate Weiss's distinctions to the different types of care distinguished in Chapter 1: physical tending, material support, psychological support, and generalized expressions of concern. Possible interrelations are shown in Figure 5.1. Physical tending, for example, may be provided by a spouse or co-residential intimate on the basis of attachment, or by kin in some circumstances as reliable assistance. It may also be provided as nurturance by a mother to a child, or a daughter to an elderly parent. Material and psychological support may similarly be derived from different sources, depending on the provisions of relationships. Generalized concern is more characteristic of people such as priests and doctors, providing guidance from respected others, or of neighbours 'keeping an eye on' people in the locality without necessarily interacting with them. The value of this cross-classification is in pointing to the complexity of motives for caring. Though framed in terms of what is delivered (as care), and the type of relationship on which it is based, it is suggestive of some of the reasons why people do provide care.

Can these be specified more precisely? Roy Parker has succinctly posed some of the questions to be asked:

What induces people to help others? What kinds of motivations operate? Are we examining transactions which are primarily economic or transactions which are social and altruistic? If they are of a mixed quality, what blend does that mixture contain?

Figure 5.1 Interrelationships in Informal Care between Types of Care and Provisions of Relationships

Provisions of relationships

Types of care	Attachment	Social integration	Nurturance	Reassurance of worth	Reliable assistance	Guidance from respected others
Physical tending	Spouse or other co-residential intimate		Daughter or mother		Kin in some circumstances	
Material support	Spouse or other co-residential intimate	Kin	Daughter or mother or sibling		Kin; neighbours	
Psychological support	Spouse or other co-residential intimate	Friends		Friends; workmates; nuclear family	Kin; neighbours	
Generalized concern					Neighbours	Priest; doctor

Taken further, what qualities do we think the tending relationship should have, and ought social policy to play a role in their
achievement? . . . What differences are introduced by payment
(to those providing care)? Have we been gently steered away
from issues concerning the social distribution of tending by the
particularly moral quality that has come to be attached to the
act of tending? (Parker, 1981, p. 30).

ALTRUISM

The moral quality to which Parker refers has been particularly
associated with altruism, commonly defined in terms such as
'regard for others as a principle of action'. One of the most
influential recent analyses of the role of altruism in social welfare
was Richard Titmuss' *The Gift Relationship* (1970), which argued
that social policy extends opportunities for altruism in contrast to
the possesive egoism of the market-place. 'The grant, or the gift,
or the unilateral transfer – whether it takes the form of cash, time,
energy, satisfaction, blood or even life itself – is the distinguishing
mark of the social (in policy and administration) just as exchange
or bilateral transfer is the mark of the economic' (Titmuss, 1968,
p. 22). He concluded his analysis of the role of giving in the
supply of blood with the words: 'Freedom from disability is
inseparable from altruism' (Titmuss, 1970, p. 246). The limitations of family, community and class could be transcended to
provide for the 'universal stranger' and it was in society's treatment of the 'universal stranger' that altruism found its fullest
expression. In modern society, more rather than less provision
needs to be made for 'the expression of altruism in the daily life of
all social groups' (Titmuss, 1970, p. 224).

Titmuss' argument is not directly generalizable to informal
social care, since he focused on the impersonal gift to the 'universal stranger', recognizing that giving in the everyday settings of
neighbourhood and community was a more complex matter
(Bulmer, 1986a, p. 104). Nevertheless, *The Gift Relationship* has
usually been read – and rightly – as a clear statement of the role of
altruism in social policy, and, by implication, the application of
that principle in areas other than that of blood donation (for one
such example see Land and Rose, 1985).

Titmuss was attempting to formulate a norm which would apply generally to social care and institutionalized social support. He was concerned with

> large areas of gift actions and behaviour in both personal and impersonal contexts which do not involve physical objects, which are difficult or impossible to price or quantify in economic terms, and which, while involving an act of giving, carry no explicit right, expectation or moral enforcement of a return gift. . . . Manifestations of altruism in this sense may of course be thought of as self-love. But they may also be thought of as giving life, or prolonging life, or enriching life for anonymous others. (Titmuss, 1970, p. 212)

The scope for altruism has most usually been discussed either in terms of the psychology of behaviour, or of the formal, bureaucratized social policy provision of the state, or in terms of the psychology and sociology of helping[1] Nevertheless the debate is highly relevant to the provision of informal care in the community by kin and non-kin on the basis of personal ties. To what extent is such care best understood as being based upon altruism?

Can such a regard of a purely selfless kind be generalized to the provision of whole areas of social care? *The Gift Relationship* has been criticized on just these grounds. It has been pointed out, for example, that although the British system of blood donation is altruistic, only a very small proportion of the population – perhaps one in twenty – actively participate in it. 'The picture of a broadly altruistic society seems somewhat blurred when we realise what a small fraction of the population is in fact functioning altruistically' (Arrow, 1972, pp. 347–8). The world supply of plasma, as opposed to whole blood, is dominated by the United States, which relies for its supply on paid donors (Drake, Finkelstein and Sapolsky, 1982; Singer, 1983). Countries such as Britain, which rely on donors for whole blood but on the market for plasma, are not as purely altruistic as Titmuss argued.

Moreover, the extent to which all British blood donors are purely selfless in their actions may be doubted. While the one-half of American donors who give blood free of charge (usually either to replace blood given to relatives or to ensure such a future right for themselves) are not regarded as behaving altruistically, the twenty-eight per cent of British donors who have themselves received transfusions or have relatives who have received transfusions are regarded as behaving altruistically. In terms of a formal calculus the distinction can probably be maintained, but in the latter case the element of long-term, diffuse recognition of some norm of reciprocity seems clear. A substantial minority of British donors are not behaving purely selflessly. Moreover, empirical examples of gift-based services are few and far between, the donation of blood apart. It can be argued that the role of volunteers within the personal social services are of this type (cf. Uttley, 1980, pp. 201–2) but, as Philip Abrams's research on neighbourhood care showed, this is a misinterpretation both of motivation and outcome (Bulmer, 1986a).

Land and Rose have recently argued for an approach to the care of one person by another as a freely chosen course of action, invoking *The Gift Relationship*. Their point that 'altruistic practices are structured into women's lives and structured out of men's' (Land and Rose, 1985, p. 93) is well-taken, and they are right to point to structural conditions which push caring on to unpaid or cheap female labour. They argue that women must be free *not* to care as well as to care, which requires the availability of good alternative services for the dependent. Whether they are correct to term the care provided by female relatives, friends and neighbours 'compulsory altruism', however, is open to doubt. Their contrast between 'compulsory altruism' and Titmuss' 'altruistic society' seems unrealistic, since arguably the basis both of much informal care and of state welfare provision does not lie in altruism at all.

Seminal though *The Gift Relationship* has been, its contrast between altruism and egoism is overdrawn. To postulate a polarity between egoism and selfishness on one side and altruism and other regarding behaviour on the other may be seriously misleading when treated as other than an ideal type. 'Egoism' and 'altruism', if unqualified, are inapplicable to the most characteristic forms of social behaviour.

> While it would seem that an egoist is a person who is incapable of friendship, an altruist is someone who is exploitable by every 'friend' and stranger, unless they also happen to be altruists; for the egoist a social life is meaningless, for the altruist it is impossible. The egoist could be likened to a black hole in the

social universe . . . while the altruist may be compared to a brightly burning star ineffectually striving to illuminate and warm a dark and limitless universe (Pinker, 1979, p. 10).

In the real world 'altruism' and 'egoism' are more likely to be interactive and conditional (cf. Pruger, 1973). Ties between family members are a good case in point. Titmuss' general contrast between egoists in the economic market and altruists inspired by the social market does not allow for forms of familial altruism which he tends to subsume under the heading 'egoism'. Indeed, relations between kin cannot be reduced to either of the two terms.

Within the family there are complex networks of interdependence and dependency involving the exercise of power between and within generations and the sexes which affect many of the elements of everyday life. These networks provide the framework within which the most important forms of mutual aid occur (Pinker, 1979, pp. 13–14).

There is an important distinction between familial and extra-familial altruism which the notion of the 'universal stranger' does not capture. Part of the difficulty arises from treating actors as isolated individuals, acting exclusively on their own behalf. In practice, of course, the majority of people are trying to act at least in the best interests of other members of their kin network, and probably also having regard to certain friends and neighbours as well. They may also have regard to the wider collective interest, for instance, in acting in such a way as to conserve natural resources, or energy, or in not smoking in certain situations to preserve other people's health. Such behaviour is not egoistic, but neither is it adequately explained by invoking the 'universal stranger'.

Does the broader social science literature throw any light on the use of the term? Psychologists, sociologists, and economists all recognize that altruism enters into social behaviour and is an important basis for social action. For Durkheim, for example, altruism was 'the fundamental basis for social life'. While recognizing the existence of both 'egotistical' and 'altruistic' conduct, in *The Division of Labour in Society* (1933) he contested the Spencerian view of society as composed of competitive individuals or the Darwinian struggle for the survival of the fittest. Durkheim pointed to what he saw as 'the essential element of moral life, that is, the moderating influence that society exercises over its members, which tempers and neutralises the brutal action of the struggle for existence and selection. Wherever there are societies, there is altruism, because there is solidarity' (1933, p. 197).

Even economists, whose theoretical models postulate egoism, self-interest and selfishness as the basis of economic behaviour, have increasingly recognized that altruism plays some role alongside market mechanisms (cf. Polanyi, 1957; Collard, 1978; Sugden, 1984). Organized philanthropy is perhaps the most obvious example (cf. Dickinson, 1962). The whole structure of government tax and expenditure involves a departure from self-interest; taxpayers must contribute to general government expenditure without knowing what proportion of their contributions they will receive back in return. The complaints of road users that taxes on vehicles and petrol are not reflected in expenditure on new roads is a case in point. Though it is doubtful whether government can be treated as an altruistic actor, is some respects its disbursements may be regarded as a form of altruism (Arrow, 1972, p. 345). A recent analysis of goodwill in relations between firms suggests that its existence may be a factor of some significance in explaining the superior economic performance of the Japanese economy (Dore, 1983). The family, as Adam Smith pointed out, is usually the closest and most personal concern of every economic actor. By extension, it has been argued by Gary Becker (1981) that altruism is more characteristic of economic behaviour in the family and selfishness of economic behaviour in the market-place.

Becker's argument (1981, Chapter 8) starts by quoting Adam Smith on self-interest in the market-place – 'It is not from the benevolence of the butcher, the brewer or the baker that we expect our dinner . . . ' – and affection as the basis of relations within the family, reinterpreting the latter by an unjustified elision as altruism. The assumptions that members of families behave altruistically to one another is nowhere justified, and although Becker develops an elegant theoretical argument from the distinction, the value of the initial distinction, both as to pure self-interest in the market-place and pure altruism in the family, must be doubted.

A more subtle economic analysis of personal ties was provided by Fred Hirsch in his discussion of the economics of bad neighbours in *Social Limits to Growth* (1977). He tied altruism firmly to relationships of attachment and intimacy, rather than to kinship ties (Becker) or an impersonal regard for the general good.

> In a deep friendship or love between two people, the mutual benefit in taking the long view rather than the short can be assumed to be sufficiently ingrained for this basis of exchange to emerge implicity. There will be sufficient trust for the implied contract of give and take to be honored and faithfully interpreted over time. But deep friendship and love are of course more than implied contracts of long-term exchange. They involve a greater or lesser degree of altruism. To put it another way, the well-being of the other partner adds directly (though not necessarily equally) to one's own, or more radically, may be integrally merged with one's own well-being (Hirsch, 1977, p. 78)

Hirsch was not alone in linking altruism to love. Becker's equation of altruism with the family (predominantly the nuclear family) comes close to doing that, though, as will be argued below, to extend the notion to kinship relations is unconvincing. Pitrim A. Sorokin, the sociologist whose later years at Harvard were devoted to fostering a Center for Creative Altruism, made the same equation in one of his main publications on the subject (1950). A commentator on Durkheim suggests that altruism is surely another name for love (Poggi, 1972, p. 240), yet it is stretching the term 'love' to suggest that all other-regarding action is of this type. The parable of the Good Samaritan is powerful and evocative, but its value is exemplary rather than as a social norm. An appeal to pure love for one's fellow men and women can hardly be the general basis of social care, either informal or formal. Hirsch at least does tie altruism to relationship of close intimacy. As Bernard Williams has pointed out, 'some of our decent actions come not from that motive which Christians misrepresent as our loving everybody, but just from our loving somebody' (Williams, 1973, p. 85).

Hirsch emphasizes, however, that other informal social relationships, for example, friendship, are characterized much more by reciprocity and mutual exchange than by altruism. Moreover, the 'economics of bad neighbours' can render such relationships decreasingly worth participating in. Assessing the costs involved, people may find other activities substantially more profitable compared to the high costs and low rewards of making friends with neighbours. While from a public point of view collective public provision is costly and reliance on informal neighbourhood care cheap, for the individual the balance of advantage is reversed. The costs of positive caring for others – whether neighbours or, more probably, kin – are very high, often exorbitant, while those of the welfare state are, for the individual at least, low, and they are anyway unavoidable through taxation. There is thus some tendency to withdraw from such informal commitments and allow public provision to bear the burden of care. (This argument also runs counter to Titmuss' view that free availability of welfare services encourages additional voluntary altruistic help – Weale, 1978, pp. 118–9.)

Certain post-war social trends encouraged these tendencies to withdrawal. Hirsch quoted Kropotkin (1904) to support the argument that withdrawal was linked to increasing affluence; mutual aid was less common among the well off than among the poor. People now placed more value on their own time, to use for leisure activities, and not for performing tasks for people they were not intimate with. Increasing geographical and social mobility reduced the probability that those whom one helped would be in a position to return the exchange.

Hirsch's argument anticipates a discussion of reciprocity and exchange theory which follows below. So far as altruism is concerned, he convincingly suggested that it was confined to relationships of attachment and intimacy – the left-hand column of Figure 5.1 on p. 147. Even here, it may be argued that there is a high degree of reciprocity in such intimate relationships, and that altruistic behaviour of one partner caring for the other is a return for services provided in the past. What seems clear, however, is that altruism cannot be convincingly adduced as the basis of other forms of relationship as set out by Robert Weiss (see pp 143–6). One must look elsewhere for a convincing explanation of why the majority of people provide informal care, without necessarily following Philip Abrams all the way in treating altruism as a form of reciprocity.

BENEFICENCE

A second principle which may be invoked to explain the provision of care, broader than altruism, is that of beneficence. Alvin Gouldner contrasted the norm of reciprocity (of which more below) with the norm of beneficence, recognizing that the former 'cannot apply with full force in relations with children, old people, or with those who are mentally or physically handicapped' (Gouldner, 1960, p. 178). The problem of the dependent, of those having nothing to offer, was solved in Gouldner's eyes by the requirement that 'people should help those who need help'. Though his main analysis emphasized the calculative relationships of reciprocity, he recognized that people must have some duties to others which are not the rights of those others. Some form of 'moral absolutism' or a norm of giving must intervene.

> The norm of beneficence calls upon men to aid others without thought of what they have done or can do for them, and solely in terms of a need imputed to the potential recipient . . . [It] is a diffuse one encompassing a number of somewhat more concrete normative orientations such as 'altruism', 'charity', or 'hospitality'. In short, the norm calls on men to give something for nothing. (Gouldner, 1973, p. 266)

Beneficence carries with it the overtones of moral authority and duty. The argument has recently been propounded that we owe special responsibilities to those who are particularly vulnerable to us, and therefore need help. One example given is that of relations between friends. Such relations may be interpreted as based on affective ties. But relations of friendship also depend upon trust, and trust entails reliance on the other person. This places upon each party to the relationship the responsibility to behave towards the other with regard to their well-being and the possible damage which could be done to them. Among friends there is mutual emotional vulnerability. If a friend lets you down, you are hurt deeply and feel betrayed.

This greater emotional vulnerability between persons who reciprocate affection explains why their responsibilities should

be reciprocal and especially strong. The obligations of friendship consist essentially in mutual consideration for the feelings
of others (Goodin, 1985, p. 98).

Goodin generalizes this argument to hold that special responsibilities follow from special vulnerabilities rather than from special self-assumed obligations.

> What gives rise to the duty to act in cases of . . . personal ties
> . . . is the state of mutual reliance that exists within such
> relationships and the dependence and helplessness of him who
> claims that the duty is owing to him. And what makes expecta-
> tions of material support particularly justifiable in intimate
> associations is the even more important emotional vul-
> nerabilities among the participants (Goodin, 1985, p. 72).

Helping the dependant does not therefore arise from pure 'goodness of heart' but from a moral recognition of the dependant's
dependency and vulnerability. A voluntaristic account in terms of
self-assumed obligations is inadequate to explain why people act
to meet the dependency needs of others.

Beneficence is also evident in charitable welfare activity, of
which one prototype was the large-scale charitable activities in
industrial areas in the middle and later nineteenth centuries,
before state welfare provision (other than the Poor Law) had
developed. Such giving by members of the upper- and upper-
middle classes was not done from purely altruistic motives but
from notions of the appropriate beneficent responsibilities of
persons in their social position. A strict sense of social hierarchy
prevailed, but such beneficence – evidenced, for example, in the
Settlement House movement – had a firm moral base. Going back
further, another example is the responsibility which upper-class
landowners recognized to care for their servants, estate workers
and tenants when ill or living in retirement, providing them with
housing and small pensions in infirmity or old age, albeit at a
fairly minimal level. Such paternalism was grounded in a strict
hierarchical and deferential social system, based on long common
residence, the foundation of which was ultimately in an acknowledged moral responsibility to behave in a beneficent way.

TRADITION

Tradition is clearly another basis on which care is provided. Traditional action is action following on from the habituation of long practice (Weber, 1947, p. 115). A number of types of caring relationships are relationships entered into for other reasons which, with the passage of time, turn into caring relationships of one sort or another. Tradition is one element, though not the only or most important one, in elderly spouses caring for each other in infirm old age. An interesting example is provided by a study done at the National Institute of Social Work of carers of the confused mentally infirm elderly (Levin, Sinclair and Gorbach, 1986). This found that a principal characteristic of supporters other than spouses (for example, siblings caring for a confused elderly person) was that they had lived together for a long time, averaging more than twenty years. Supporters were as likely to be members of the same generation as the confused elderly person, as they were to be of the younger generation of adult children. This applied not only to spouses but to siblings; the longest time found living together was seventy-four years, dating from the day that the supporter, a sister, had been born. Even among supporters who belonged to a younger generation, average length of residence together with the person cared for was over fifteen years, accounted for mainly by sons and daughters, singly or in pairs, who had always lived with their parents. Similarly, studies of care between neighbours suggest that the longer someone has lived in a particular area, the greater likelihood there is of their receiving support from their co-residents (Bulmer, 1986a).

As noted in Chapter 1, 'community care' is a resonant term because it embodies within it some of the attributes of beneficence and tradition. The term 'community' in this context invokes implicity what Walzer calls 'communities of character, historically stable origin, associations of men and women with some special commitment to one another and some special sense of their common life' (Walzer 1981, p. 32). The notion of 'community care' has implicit in it the idea that special duties are owed to members of one's own community, over more general duties or obligations one may have to larger collectivities. The difficulty of the term, as we have seen, is whether empirically such communities exist and whether the nature of people's attachment to place is such that it leads to recognition of such special duties. The term 'community care' invokes 'communities of character', when empirically their existence is problematical. To the extent that they do exist (for example, in rural villages (cf. Bulmer, 1986a, pp. 63–71)) tradition plays a very important element in strengthening the ties through which care is provided.

DUTY OR OBLIGATION

Distinct from tradition, but having some affinity with it and with beneficence, is care provided through a sense of duty or obligation. Such ideas are very important in understanding why people provide social care, and do not generally receive enough attention. The contrasts drawn earlier between kinship, friendship and neighbouring ties brought out the special obligatory character of kinship relations. Kin relations are ties that are inescapable – one is born with them and retains them until one's death. In rare circumstances they may be modified legally (as in adoption) or informally (as in the institution of fictive kinship among black families – Malson, 1982, pp. 42–43), but they are ascribed social characteristics which are with one always. Whether or not particular kinship ties are invested with content is an empirical matter, but the fact of their existence entails a presumptive obligation.

The recognition of kinship obligations is an ancient one. Consider the English lawyer, W. Blackstone, in the eighteenth century on the responsibilities of children to their aged parents:

> They, who protected the weakness of our infancy, are entitled to our protection in the infirmity of their age; they who by sustenance and education have enabled their offspring to prosper, ought in return to be supported by that offspring in case they stand in need of assistance. Upon this principle proceed all the duties of children to their parents. (Blackstone, 1783, Book 1, Chapter 16)

There are a variety of types of behaviour into which obligation and duty enter as considerations. There is, moreover, a distinction between actions undertaken out of a sense of duty, and those which exceed the expectations of ordinary citizens (Urmson, 1969, p. 68). A good deal of mutual aid – both within and outside the family – is of the former type, and is not usefully treated as 'altruism'. In discussing the relative benevolence shown between firms in the Japanese textile industry, not pushing sub-contractors too hard in times of recession, Dore (1983) suggests that the underlying reason for this type of behaviour stems from a sense of duty. A particular sense of diffuse obligation to the individual trading partner leads to firms modifying profit-maximzing behaviour to safeguard trading partners in a weaker position at a particular point in time.

The prime example of duty and obligation in the world of informal social care is that of female relatives as carers, particularly grown-up daughters taking responsibility for elderly relatives. This issue has received a great deal of attention from social scientists in the recent past (cf. Finch and Groves, 1980; Finch and Groves, 1983; Wilson, 1982; Gamarnikov et al. 1983) and will not be discussed at length here. It is clear that many female kin consider that they have an overriding obligation to care for, or contribute to the care of, elderly parents, either by regular visiting or in certain circumstances having their parents live with them in their own home. This sense of duty or obligation is derived from the kin tie and a belief that women are particularly suited to perform caring tasks.

It is worth dwelling for a moment upon why this belief is so widely held. Weiss pointed to nurturance as one of the main provisions of social relationships, and the bond between mother and child is a particularly close one. Nels Noddings (1984) has recently traced the ethical roots of care of elderly parents by their children to the bond between mother and child. She argues that this first caring relationship (for the child) provides a model for all others. It is not contractual but of a special kind, rooted in human intuitions and feelings. Human beings carry with them the memories of, and longing for, caring and being cared for, derived from the relationship of mother and child. This caring is not a one-way process, but one in which the child actively responds, and stores up basic experiences and ethical obligations which may emerge later as apparently purely 'altruistic' or 'other regarding' behaviour.

Feminist sociologists have placed considerable emphasis upon the social subordination of women to explain why the burden of caring falls upon them. This is undoubtedly a partial explanation but it is incomplete. The caring relationship also has a moral dimension, bound up with what it is to be a woman, as Carol Gilligan has argued.

> Women's deference [to men] is rooted not only in their social subordination but also in the substance of their moral concern. Sensitivity to the needs of others and the assumption of responsibility for taking care lead women to attend to voices other than their own and to include in their judgement other points of view. Women's moral weakness, manifest in an apparent diffusion and confusion of judgement, is thus inseparable from women's moral strength, an overriding concern with relationships and responsibilities. The reluctance to judge may itself be indicative of the care and concern for others that infuse the psychology of women's development and are responsible for what is generally seen as problematic in its nature. Thus women not only define themselves in a context of human relationship, but also judge themselves in terms of their ability to care. (Gilligan, 1982, pp. 16–17)

There has tended to be a split between the possession of instrumental abilities by men – the capacity for autonomous thinking, clear decision-making and responsible action – and of expressive attributes by women – to be 'nurturer, caretaker and helpmate, the weaver of those networks of relationships' through which caring is developed (Gilligan, 1982, p. 17).

Gilligan shows that the tendency to treat women's special knowledge of relationships and care as a function of 'anatomy coupled with destiny' directs attention away from the extent to which they are an integral part of women's moral development and the definition of the appropriate goals and values for men and women, respectively. If women's moral development centres on the activity of care, derived from the understanding of responsibility and relationships, then it can be less easily fitted into male-centred theories of moral development. The point of this excursion into the moral basis of obligation to care is to emphasize the point that who are considered the appropriate carers, and who define themselves as such, is not a matter of biology or 'nature' but is socially constructed. The value of the insights of Noddings and Gilligan lies in recognizing the centrality of the nurturant relationship as the basis for the obligation to care. More worryingly for some feminists, they also suggest that there are distinctively female spheres and activities, albeit socially defined ones, and that there may be limits to the malleability of male and female social roles. The 'different voice' to which Gilligan alludes is indeed different. What is needed is more explicit recognition of the quality of that voice and its implications for social responsibilities, not the search for an androgynous substitute.

Coupled to this is needed a more thorough-going understanding of the social consequences of the definition of caring and women's work, and the social construction of obligation which is thereby entailed. Policy discussions of community care by government have been singularly deficient in ignoring the heavy burdens which caring places upon those involved in 'tending' in particular. There is now a growing awareness of the need to 'care for the carers' (cf. EOC, 1982), without any very fundamental questioning of who is doing the caring. As the discussion of 'sharing care' in the next chapter suggests, when care by informal carers becomes too burdensome, the most likely outcome is that responsibility will be transferred to the formal sector, rather than any genuine sharing taking place between the two sectors. This reflects the fact that there are limits to obligation and duty. In some circumstances, at least, 'should parents, siblings or distant kin fall upon hard times, we are increasingly inclined to say – both morally and legally – that they should lodge their claims with the state welfare services rather than with their families' (Goodin, 1985, p. 71).

RECIPROCITY

Altruism, beneficence, tradition and obligation or duty have all been considered as bases for informal care, and have been found to cover some cases of relationships based on attachment, nurturance or reliable assistance. As general explanations of why informal care is provided they are not particularly convincing, and in particular throw relatively little light upon the provisions of social integration or of reliable assistance between non-kin. The most convincing general explanation of the nature of caring relationships is to be found in terms of reciprocity, in explaining both the nature of certain ties and the caring relationships based on them. Reciprocity, for instance, clearly enters into several of the examples already discussed. Paternalist benevolence by a landowner to his tenants is in part recognition of their devotion to his service and his interests; it is not merely based upon a moral conception of responsibility. Blackstone's definition of the duties of children to elderly parents quoted on p. 158 is a description of a reciprocal relationship. And Noddings' conception of the moral basis of care rests on the reciprocal return which the child gives as an adult for the care received from its mother when a child.

Studies of reciprocity by social scientists begin with studies of primitive exchange. Where exchange took the form of reciprocal gifts rather than economic transactions, the giving of gifts was governed by a quite different morality from that of the economic market, having a multi-dimensional meaning which combined social, religious, utilitarian, sentimental, jural and moral elements.

The anthropologist Bronislaw Malinowski, in his studies of the Tropbriand Islands, was one of the first to show the importance of such reciprocity. 'The whole tribal life is permeated by a constant give and take' (Malinowski, 1922, p. 167). Malinowski emphasized that the widespread exchange of gifts was evidence of a deep-seated tendency to create social ties in this way (Malinowski, 1922, p. 175). He suggested a typology of transfers of goods, which ranged from pure gifts, through customary payments repaid irregularly, payments for services rendered, gifts returned in economically equivalent form, ceremonial barter with deferred payment, and trade, pure and simple. The classic instance of ceremonial barter was the Kula ring, a system of exchanging goods of great symbolic value within a 'ring' of Melanesian islands. Necklaces (*soulava*) circulated in a clockwise direction, armshells (*mwali*) in an anti-clockwise direction. Exchange took place between established Kula partners, with public ceremonial, in which *soulava* were exchanged for *mwali*, or vice versa. Though this is the best known of the Tropbriand exchange institutions, Malinowski's analysis of other forms of exchange are perhaps of even greater interest. In relation to payment for services rendered, for example, he remarks on the universality and strictness of the idea that

> every social obligation or duty, though it may not on any account be evaded, has yet to be repaid by a ceremonial gift. The function of these ceremonial repayments is to thicken the social ties from which arise the obligations. (Malinowski, 1922, p. 182)

The analysis of these types of exchange in primitive societies was generalized in Marcel Mauss's *The Gift,* first published in 1925. Mauss drew on a variety of ethnographic examples, including the Kula ring and the Potlatch of Indians of the Pacific North-West, to suggest a general theory of social exchange in which gifts appearing to be voluntary were in fact exchanged ceremonially as a way of forming alliances linking potentially hostile groups. On this larger political stage, reciprocity did not so much make friends as prevent hostilities breaking out. The network of alliances created thus helped to ensure a degree of political stability in societies without a stable system of rank or institutionalized means of succession. What appeared to be gifts of a disinterested kind were in fact part of elaborate systems of reciprocal exchange in which there was a delicate balance between giving and receiving. What might appear to be altruistic behaviour was in fact part of a system of mutual exchange.

Different types of reciprocity have more recently been distinguished by the American anthropologist Marshall Sahlins, who also argues that the notion of 'balance' can be overplayed. Reciprocity, in fact, is often not an unconditional one-for-one exchange, and by examining departures from balanced exchanges one understands better the interplay between reciprocity and social relations.

> Reciprocity is a whole class of exchanges, a continuum of forms . . . At one end of the spectrum stands the assistance freely given, the small currency of everyday kinship, friendship and neighbourly relations. . . . At the other pole, self-interested seizure, appropriation by chicanery or force. . . . The intervals between them . . . are intervals of sociability.

The distance between poles of reciprocity is, among other things, social distance. (Sahlins, 1965, pp. 143–4)

Sahlins distinguishes the two extremes of the continuum and a midpoint. His discussion explicitly recalls Malinowski's distinction of the six types of transaction between barter and pure gift. Sahlins sees the spirit of exchange swinging from disinterested concern for the other through mutuality to self-interest.

Generalized reciprocity represents the solidary extreme, referring to situations where the expectation of direct return is unseemly and, at best, implicit. Such transactions are 'putatively altruistic', or 'weak reciprocity' by reason of the vagueness of the obligation to reciprocate. A good indication of generalized reciprocity is a sustained one-way flow of goods or services, which does not dry up if there is no return flow. This is one extreme, apparently exemplified, for instance, by a neighbour providing material and psychological support for an elderly person.

Between the two extremes is *balanced reciprocity*, which refers to direct and equal exchange. Reciprocation is the customary equivalent of the thing received and is without delay, or after a set interval. Balanced reciprocity is less personal than generalized reciprocity. 'The pragmatic test of balanced reciprocity becomes an inability to tolerate one-way flows; the relations between people are disrupted by a failure to reciprocate within limited time and equivalence leeways' (Sahlins, 1965, p. 148). An example would be friendship, and a test of the strains imposed when one party becomes more dependent and cannot fully reciprocate as previously in the relationship.

At the other extreme is *negative reciprocity,* the attempt to get something for nothing with impunity, through several forms of appropriation. This is the most impersonal form of exchange in which the participants confront each other representing opposed interests.

Sahlins' formulation is helpful because it takes account of inequality between people and the possible extent of the need of the weaker person. Mauss used language drawn from the law of contract, and treated the obligation to give, to receive and to reciprocate as a form of contract. In generalized reciprocity, Sahlins recognized that 'the time and worth of reciprocation are not alone conditional on what was given by the donor, but also upon what he will need and when, and likewise what the recipient can afford and when' (Sahlins, 1965, p. 147). One variable influencing outcome is social distance. The closer the distance between two persons, the closer to generalized reciprocity the relationship would be. Since many personal ties are of a close, affective kind, many types of care (such as 'altruism' between close kin) may be provided on this basis. Many of the provisions of relationship discussed at the beginning of this chapter fall somewhere on the continuum between generalized and balanced reciprocity. Where kin are concerned, the relationship may move further toward negative reciprocity, to the extent that the dependent person expects care to be provided as a right or duty, contrary to the inclinations of the person providing the care.

These insights have been developed and broadened by sociologists, notably Alvin Gouldner and Philip Abrams. Gouldner showed how reciprocity enlisted egoistic motives for social purposes. Reciprocity rested on two basic principles: (1) people should help those who had helped them (2) people should not injure those who had helped them. Gouldner further distinguished between homeomorphic reciprocity (in which exchanges were identical in form) or heteromorphic reciprocity, where the things exchanged were concretely different but were regarded by the parties as equivalent. (Thus, for example, in Wenger's study, 1984, of the elderly in North Wales, dependent persons regarded help from their daughter as reciprocity for present or past child care of their grandchildren.) Thus the distinctive nexus of rights and obligations develops which is the essence of reciprocity – X and Y both owe benefits to each other and are entitled to receive benefits from each other, even though these may not be of the same type.

Philip Abrams built upon Gouldner's work and extended it considerably to encompass a discussion of altruism. He came to the view that altruism as action done for no reward ceased to be a useful way of looking at informal care. The norm of beneficence cloaked actual generalized reciprocity.

The separateness of altruism and reciprocity in principle begins to collapse in practice. Once one recognises the possibility of indirect, transferred, delayed returns one can hardly remain committed to the view that action that looks as though it is done for no reward, or action that is described subjectively as being done for no reward, is really either unrewarded or unrelated to debts incurred previously or elsewhere. The question of the possibility of an extended subterranean chain of reciprocity is bound to arise. . . . As a result reciprocity can look like beneficence at the moment it is enacted. Exchanges over time can replace exchanges now; giving to third parties can replace a direct return to a beneficiary one is unable to help directly. Having once received something for nothing from one person, one can be obliged later to give something for nothing to another. And so forth. When so many people explain their helpfulness to others in terms of the helpfulness of their own mothers such ideas are bound to be persuasive (P. Abrams in Bulmer, 1986a, p. 112).

It is arguable that Abrams exaggerated when he suggested that the psychic satisfaction derived from doing good to others was a form of return to carers, or altruism-as-reciprocity, and so rendered the relationship a reciprocal one. But there are warrants for this, the notion of self-reward encompasses similar behaviour. Psychoanalytic theory has long maintained that people may behave altruistically to avoid guilt or anxiety, or to conform to an internalized ideal, and it can be argued that people may engage in any act to gain self-reward (Hoffman, 1981, p. 134). Gary Becker in discussing the economics of the family (1981) invokes the notion of 'psychic income' as a return for certain behaviour, which is an analogous idea. Lawrence Becker (1986), a philosopher, suggests that non-voluntary social obligations are grounded in the basic moral virtue of reciprocity. Arguably the notion of reciprocity can be pushed a shade too far. Abrams' points about the long-term nature of reciprocity are, however, very well taken. Whether one calls it reciprocity or indebtedness (cf. Frankfurter, Smith and Caro, 1981), the idea of a lifetime balance-sheet of social care, particularly for members of the nuclear family, is not an inappropriate one.

At the other extreme, the argument for paying informal carers, considered in the next chapter, rests on a recognition that care is typically provided on a reciprocal basis. Among black single parents dependent upon welfare, a mutual support system is created, based on fictive kinship, through which mutual aid is provided. Among the urban working class this is comparatively unusual, and there is more scope for involving neighbours and others in the care of the dependent. Where such carers themselves have relatively low incomes, and particularly where they are not personally known to those they are caring for, there is a strong argument for payment for services rendered. This is a form of reciprocity.

As a further extension of this approach, social exchange theory has been employed to explain the nature of reciprocity in informal care. Titmuss' distinction in principle between the grant or gift as the distinguishing mark of the social compared to exchange or bilateral transfer as the mark of the economic is decisively rejected as a guide to policy for informal care. 'Most often, social policy transactions are erroneously conceived in ideal or pure terms, bearing little or no resemblance to economic or market exchange. In reality, however, the vast majority of all transactions, economic and social, occur on a continuum between these theoretical poles' (Pruger, 1973, p. 289).

Theories of 'social exchange' or 'rational choice' draw on an analogy with economic exchange but apply to the broader social realm (cf. Homans, 1961; Blau, 1964; Heath, 1976). They also draw on anthropological studies of the gift, for 'the exchange of gifts and favours between friends, neighbours and kin are strong and enduring threads in the social fabric' (Heath, 1976, p. 1). Outside the market one finds that 'neighbours exchange favours; children, toys; colleagues, assistance; acquintances, courtesies; politicians, concessions; discussants, ideas; housewives, recipes' (Blau, 1964, p. 88).

One of the main proponents of social exchange theory, Peter Blau, suggested that two features were central. Reciprocity was involved. At the same time, there was an appearance of disinterested generosity. Social exchange differed from economic exchange in that although a return was expected this involved 'diffuse future obligations, not precisely specified ones, and the nature of the return cannot be bargained about but must be left to the discretion of the one who makes it' (Blau, 1964, p. 93). Self-interest would lead to reciprocation of gifts received, and thereby feelings of gratitude and trust would be engendered.

The general form of the theory is of less interest than its application to informal care. The most explicit use of exchange theory has been by Michael Anderson. In his study of family structure in nineteenth-century Lancashire he used exchange theory to explain patterns of mutual support in the family when faced with sickness, death or unemployment. Though neighbours could provide help, they lacked a firm enough base of reciprocation in a heterogeneous and mobile society.

> Kinship, by contrast, could provide this structured link, and could thus form a basis for reciprocation. Kin did, indeed, probably provide the main source of aid. However, because this was a poor (and also a rapidly changing) society this aid . . . was limited in cost, and family and kinship relationships tended to have strong, short-run instrumental overtones of a calculative kind (Anderson, 1971, p. 171).

This interpretation has been contested on the basis of New England data by T. K. Hareven, who argues that, while this model may explain short-run routine exchanges, it does not account for long-term kin assistance with few visible rewards.

> Young family members who subordinated their own careers to family needs did so out of a sense of responsibility, affection and familial obligation rather than with the expectation of eventual gain. Within this context, kin assistance was not strictly calculative. Rather it expressed an overall principle of reciprocity over the life course (Hareven, 1982, p. 108).

What this historical controversy clearly brings out is the point insisted upon by Malinowski in relation to primitive economy; that strict exchange and social reciprocity are not the same. Social reciprocity is a broader category, in which although there is recognition of mutual obligation it may be extended in time and somewhat uncertain as to the return to be received. An appreciation of this point is essential to grasp the nature of informal social care.

Other studies of informal care which draw on exchange theory are Philip Abrams's studies of neighbouring (Bulmer, 1986a) and Wellman's studies of support networks, where he treats the social system as networks of dependency relationships resulting from the differential possession of scare resources at the nodes and the structured allocation of these resources at the ties. Such ties are often asymmetrically reciprocal, differing in content and intensity. But 'while ties are rarely symmetric, they are usually reciprocated in a generalised way' (Wellman, 1983, p. 172).

An interesting use of the theory is in Hazel Qureshi's analysis of the motivations of carers and clients in the Kent Community Care scheme. This was an experimental project to give locally based social workers control of a budget to buy goods and services to tailor care to clients' individual needs. The scheme involved the extensive recruitment of local people as helpers, either unpaid or paid pocket-money for their contribution (Challis and Davies, 1980). Those clients who were aware whether their helpers were paid or unpaid definitely preferred them to be paid. However, 'it was also clear that, once a warm relationship was established, clients wanted to be sure that helpers did not come just for the money. Exchange theory suggests that there is no inconsistency here. The payments made to the helpers by a third party enable the client to feel that there is a balance of benefits in the exchange. Hence there is no requirement for the client to feel deference or gratitude' (Qureshi, Challis and Davies, 1983, p. 165). Despite their dependent situation, a number of carers also made efforts to reciprocate the help given to them by the helpers. One of Qureshi's conclusions has particularly important policy implications for the provision of informal care:

> The use of the social exchange framework . . . in particular . . . suggests that, where there is no pre-existing relationship, it may be an advantage rather than a disadvantage, in building up a relationship with the elderly person, for the helper to be paid (Qureshi, 1985, p. 9).

The Kent research provided evidence about the motivations of helpers. In relation to the present discussions, although about three-quarters of helpers referred to altruistic motivations for their actions, many of them had quite instrumental reasons for getting involved in the scheme, such as filling their time, earning a little money, or using their involvement as a stepping-stone to work in the social services field. Even when their motivation appeared to be purely altruistic, in some cases it was self-interested altruism (Arrow, 1972), in the sense that the helpers gained satisfaction not only from helping the clients but from the knowledge that they themselves had helped to bring about a change. In many cases a mixture of motives appeared to operate, so that it was difficult to distil out a pure form of altruism. Tradition also played a part. Those who referred to helping as 'A natural instinct' or 'It's just something in me', had had experience of helping, most as nurses working at the time the survey took place, or previously. How far such responses reflect this pattern of work experience and the ideology of the nursing profession as a whole is hard to judge, but clearly past experience played some part in the type of explanations offered.

Motivational explanations clearly need to be treated with circumspection. Neighbourhood care schemes, for example, may fulfil other purposes than those stated by the participants. The Abrams team found a striking example of a scheme devoted to visiting and transporting the elderly whose latent function appeared to be to provide congenial social activity for the helpers (Bulmer, 1986a, pp. 156–8, 199–200). Studies of the motives of volunteers have shown that it is notoriously difficult to pinpoint accurately the reasons for participation in voluntary work (cf. Qureshi, Davies and Challis, 1979). Diana Leat suggests a shift in strategy to stop asking questions about motivation, which easily become bogged down in esoteric arguments about 'real' and 'underlying' motives.

> Instead, it may be more illuminating to ask about the expectations of, and rewards derived from, different types of volunteering, and to relate these to the volunteer's personal and social circumstances and the perceived alternative courses of action available to such a volunteer (Leat, 1983b, p. 52).

Such an approach in terms of expectations and rewards directs attention naturally toward reciprocity and the exchange element in the caring relationship.

Nor does 'concern for others' provide an adequate explanation of why people volunteer (cf. Hadley, Webb and Farrell, 1976). To achieve such an explanation one has to compare volunteers with non-volunteers, and look at the type of means chosen to help people, for example, participation in a formal scheme versus informal neighbouring. When one looks at such means, certain patterns emerge. For instance, it is notably the case that middle-class volunteers tend to get involved in formal helping, while working-class volunteers tend to be more involved in informal helping. The Abrams *et al.* national study of 'good neighbour' schemes (1981) found that availability was inversely related to the need for such schemes, the main explanation of which was the social class composition of the areas from which the volunteers were drawn. Beside this finding, of course, needs to be set the fact that one of the most effective groups of paid carers, home helps, are drawn almost entirely from the working class and that they look after the needs of a largely, though not exclusively, working-class clientele.

There are no straightforward answers to the question of why people care for one another. It is quite clear, however, that the polar ideal types of egoism and altruism, of pure, self-centred self-interest on the one hand and pure, other-regarding behaviour on the other, are of very limited usefulness in understanding patterns of caring. Beneficence, obligation and duty, and tradition all play some part in explaining why people behave as they do. The most adequate theoretical approach, however, is in terms of the reciprocity and social exchanges involved in the provision of informal social care.

To sum up, these reflections upon the philosophical and sociological bases of caring underline the extent to which informal caring grows out of existing social relationships. It is not something to be 'engineered' in a mechanical way, for example, by 'upholding' or 'plugging in' to networks. This has major implications for an important theme pursued in the next chapter, the possibilities for arranging substitute carers. To the extent that care rests upon reciprocity, this implies the existence of continuing relationships in the past. How one carer or supporter is substituted for another has to take account of those relationships, and explains, for example, why in Figure 5.1 on p. 147, the range of informal carers available to undertake physical tending is so limited.

NOTES

1   On the first of these see Krebs, 1970; Macaulay and Berkowitz, 1970. On the second see Pruger, 1973; Uttley, 1980. On the third see Friedrichs, 1960; Weiner, 1976; Lenrow, 1978; Rushton and Sorrentino, 1981.

6

Interweaving Formal and Informal Care

Many policy dilemmas for 'community care' appear with greatest clarity when one examines the possibility of linking formal and informal care. Such policies currently have a high profile. The Barclay Report of 1982 placed great emphasis on harnessing informal social networks. In September 1984 the Secretary of State for Social Services spoke of a new role for Social Service departments, not just in delivering statutory services but in co-ordinating services provided by themselves, voluntary agencies and the private sector (*The Guardian*, 28 September 1984; Bulmer, 1986c). The increasing attention paid to informal care has encouraged policy-makers to think of ways of making statutory and non-statutory services complementary to one another, with the particular aim of postponing the need for residential or institutional care for as long as possible. In mental handicap and mental illness provision, the reverse policy of decanting institutional populations into 'the community' also depends on the ability to mobilize various forms of informal care.

FORMAL AND INFORMAL CARE

Care, as noted in Chapter 1, may be provided by statutory, voluntary, private for-profit sources, or informally by kin, neighbours and friends, 'natural' helpers and self-help and mutual aid activities. Over-simplifying, formal caring relationships are relationships of *gesellschaft* while informal caring relationships are relationships of *gemeinschaft*. Formal care in this chapter refers to statutory, voluntary or private commercial provision for social care. All statutory social services are formal welfare institutions, in that they are governed by explicit rules defining their objectives and management. Parts of the voluntary sector are also formal institutions, with explicit rules, paid and, in some cases, professionally-qualified staff. Many voluntary organizations are also dependent upon government funding, which gives them a more formal status (Pinker, 1985, p. 106). Whether paid or not, volunteers are usually part of formal organizations pursing specified objectives within a framework of rules. The private sector is also run on rational, instrumental lines, and is subject to government regulation and fiscal requirements which constitute a framework of rules. In the United States, the lines separating the voluntary, private market and government provision of care are even less sharp than in Britain (Froland, 1980, p. 585, n. 4).

The scope of informal care will be clear from preceding chapters. It refers to care based on personal ties where the person receiving care is treated as an end in themselves and receives help on the basis of some kind of personal relationship, not for instrumental reasons (such as the performance of a job). Usually such caring activities are unorganized and spontaneous.

The distinction is a conceptual one. It can be effectively applied to most empirical instances, but there is a borderline between formal and informal care which constitutes a grey area. Consider the following examples. A clergyman visiting housebound parishioners is ostensibly providing formal support, since these duties are part of his calling. Yet, if he has been a minister in one place for a long period he will very likely have developed personal ties with members of his flock. Similarly, the home help who is paid to provide household assistance to the elderly and housebound but who does additional tasks for the client in time which is not paid for, because of affective ties to that person, in a sense also straddles the line. Clients, too, develop such attachments. 'I don't call her "Home Warden" or "Mrs", I call her Alice and she's my angel' (Bulmer, 1986a, p. 212). 'Good neighbour' schemes, described by Philip Abrams as cheshire cat organizations which come into existence only to try to make themselves disappear (Abrams *et al.*, 1981) also exist on the boundary between the informal and the formal, trying to formalize the informal or to foster the informal out of the formal. Some mutual aid schemes, such as Alcoholics Anonymous, have developed from modest informal beginnings into large voluntary organizations, straddling the divide over time.

For practical purposes it is useful to confine informal care mainly to care between kin, neighbours and friends, and to treat as formal care care undertaken within some external organization (however loose that organization may be – such as a neighbourhood care group). It is also useful to treat as formal care voluntary care where there is some accountability to an intermediary (Gilroy, 1982, p. 13). Once the distinction is clear, the relationship between the two types of care has to be conceptualized. Here, the most frequently used metaphors are those of complementarity or a continuum, or the simile of 'interweaving'.

Michael Bayley, after introducing the distinction between care *in* and care *by* the community, set out the case for a partnership between statutory social services on the one hand and informal care by families, friends and neighbours on the other.

> The social services seek to interweave their help so as to use and strengthen the help already given, make good the limitations and meet the needs. It is not a question of the social services plugging the gaps but rather of their working with *society* to enable *society* to close the gaps. (Bayley, 1973, p. 343)

In this view, formal and informal care are complementary to one another. Other scholars have formulated the complementarity in terms of a continuum between informal and more intimate support to formal and institutional support.

> At the informal end are personal needs involving affectual relationships, emotional interaction, intellectual stimulation. Straddling informal and formal are needs for personal and physical maintenance, such as washing, toileting, moving about, eating etc. A little further on is the need for housing, the need to be productive, and ultimately the need for full security

in terms of specialised medical and rehabilitative services, residential care, and for total income support (Graycar, 1983, p. 385).

Different services are seen as meeting different types of need in a mutually supportive fashion.

Yet this view was not without its critics, such as Philip Abrams in Britain (Bulmer, 1986a, pp. 208–19) and Charles Froland in the United States. Froland suggested 'a view of the relationship between the formal and informal sectors of care as being less one of a continuum of compatibility and more one fraught with discontinuities and contradictions in its underlying assumptions and features' (Froland, 1980, p. 574). Philip Abrams started out his research on neighbourhood care suggesting that 'this notion of a continuum of caring relationships is in fact misleading and dangerous . . . we ought instead to start out by envisaging a discontinuity, a principled anthithesis almost between the formal and the informal' (Abrams, 1978b, p. 2). Elsewhere, he postulated the existence of a 'frontier' between the two. There was a marked difference, he argued, between bureaucratically administered services provided in a locality on the one hand, and effective informal caring by local residents on the other – 'discovering, unleashing, supporting and relying upon indigenous caring agents and locally-rooted helping networks' (Abrams, 1980, p. 13). The two types of care might, in principle, be incompatible, because they were based upon two opposed modes of social organizations: the bureaucratic and the communal.

INTERWEAVING IN PRACTICE

The idea of a continuum of care, or of 'interweaving', is thus by no means taken for granted and has been openly challenged. What happens in practice, and does practice provide pointers to the resolution of the argument between the advocates and the critics? In Britain, the general trend is clear. There is increasing interest on the part of Social Service departments in interweaving formal and informal care, and steps have been taken in that direction since the early 1970s. A variety of schemes exist to promote it. Domiciliary provision has been increased, and some authorities employ 'street wardens' to complement the home help service and provide visiting and shopping help. Some authorities have recruited volunteers, originally strangers, to act as visitors to the housebound and dependent. 'Good neighbour' schemes (Abrams *et al.*, 1981) have been funded in some cases by local authorities. More support services have been provided for mentally handicapped and mentally ill patients discharged from hospital, some of them linked to informal care. Some social work teams have put greater emphasis on the complementary of statutory and non-statutory provision, focused either upon specific client groups (such as the elderly mentally infirm) or upon specific localities, as in 'patch' services provided in small, local areas aimed at all types of client.

Such developments have been uneven and, despite the interest on the part of DHSS ministers in broadening the responsibilities of Social Service departments, in some areas have not gone very far in this direction. There is still much 'separate development' of formal and informal services, as the following example of alternation between the two types of care shows.

> An elderly mentally infirm person would typically live alone or with a frail spouse, receiving regular help from other family members and occasional help from old friends or neighbours, some of whom might visit under the wing of the local neighbourhood care scheme. A home help might visit twice a week, and a hot lunch might be delivered three days a week. As things become more serious, pressure would be put on a relative other than a spouse to take on full-time care. A daughter might give up a paid job and astonishingly, once the old person moves in with her and her family, all domiciliary services could be withdrawn. After a year, the unsupported relative would be unable to tolerate the intensity of 365 days a year caring for her infirm parent and would refuse to provide care any longer, probably in a mood of acute guilt and distress. The elderly person would move with great suddenness from the informal world to the statutory, entering full-time residential care either in a local-authority home or a psychogeriatric ward, depending on the severity of his mental impairment (Darvill, 1983, pp. 243–4).

Informal care is clearly of key importance, and cannot be

dispensed with. Informal care-givers remain the first point of reference for people seeking help. An individual's social network is the reference point for seeking and obtaining help in the first instance, and the help provided is generally effective in meeting that person's immediate needs. There are good reasons why such personal ties are the best basis for providing care: informal carers can respond immediately to crises, can provide everyday assistance, offer emotional reassurance, and supply long-term care of a straightforward kind. Professionally trained personnel are not well able to cope with events that are unpredicatable, where there are too many contingencies or where tasks are not easily subdivided. Such conditions are basic to everyday life, and being non-uniform, are managed most effectively by primary group members (Litwak, 1985, pp. 10–11).

Informal care, however, has a number of limitations. The coverage provided by informal care is uneven, depending as it does on personal ties and the density of the social networks in which the individual is located. Estimates vary, but as many as one-quarter of elderly people may have no close relatives to whom they can turn for help. Informal networks may be strong in one area, weak in another. Even in an area with strong networks, the individual with no relatives or friends may be isolated (see Chapter 3). There are considerable variations in the strength of ties between people living in the same locality, and differing conceptions of the responsibilities of neighbours to one another. Even if personal ties as the basis of care exist, there are problems in ensuring continuity of care among kin, neighbours and friends. As the mental handicap example shows, burdens may become too great, but even if they do not, personal circumstances and inclinations may vary, affecting what they can offer to the person cared for.

A prime circumstance in which professional help is needed is where the informal carer lacks sufficient skills or knowledge to deal with the problem concerned, as in the classic instance of medical problems requiring treatment by a doctor or nurse. The same may be true of someone suffering physical impairment such as blindness, deafness, or stiffness of the limbs, requiring specialist advice on the handicap or treatment to deal with it (such as physiotherapy). Mental illness may require the services of a psychiatrist or community psychiatric nurse. Continuing professional care may not be required once diagnosis is made, but if a condition is changing then regular professional monitoring may be required. The skills possessed by social workers are more diffuse than those of medical personnel, but may be of critical importance, for example, in assessing the social circumstances and ability to cope with an elderly person being discharged from hospital.

Professional care is also appropriate in exceptional or unusual circumstances. The most obvious of these is statutory responsibility for child care. The state (through local authority Social Service departments) has a duty to intervene if it is suspected that children are being ill-treated by their parents. In some circumstances, children may be separated from their parents and taken into local authority residential or foster-care if their parents are unable to cope or they themselves are judged to be at risk. Professional involvement may also be most appropriate for people whose problems are not necessarily ones they would wish to share with friends or neighbours, such as being a one-parent family in difficult financial circumstances, or looking after a mentally handicapped child, or suffering from alcoholism, or from personal psychological difficulties. Considerations of personal privacy discussed in Chapter 3 may suggest formal care is more appropriate in such circumstances for 'informal networks may be experienced as oppressive, or even vindictive, and the "sufferer" may feel he is the object of idle yet hurtful gossip rather more than the subject of genuine care and concern. Often the very last people those with such problems would go to for help would be their neighbours or friends' (Gilroy, 1982, p. 14). Finally, a different reason for formal provision may be to ensure equity of treatment for certain types of case. A classic, if paradoxical, example, is compulsory education from the ages of 5 to 16. The state intervenes to say that all children *must* attend school, and it enforces this rule if necessary.

Many of the types of care being considered could potentially be provided either by formal or informal carers. Moreover, the line drawn between is not always clear cut. 'The edges are blurred, and the informal can humanize and sensitize the formal while the formal can stimulate and support the informal' (Bayley, 1982, p. 181). The home help service is an excellent example of a service which falls into this category, where there is indeed a degree of substitutability between the formal and informal sectors. Studies of home help provision have repeatedly shown that old people who live alone receive more help than people who live with their families. Living alone is used as a convenient criterion for priority allocation, regardless of the exact circumstances of the elderly person. The policy problem is what level of support to provide for the family which is doing the caring. In Britain it seems to be feared that if the state assumes too many responsibilities families will abrogate their caring role toward kin, but there is also recognition that if the state offers too little help the family may collapse under the unrelieved burden (Land and Parker, 1978). Sharing care involves making quite fine judgements about the extent to which people receive support from informal sources.

Within Social Services departments, home help services tend to be fairly self-contained functions. There is relatively little input, for example, from social workers (Dexter and Harbert, 1983, p. 168). A majority of clients are referred direct to organizers without social work intervention, many of them by doctors or nurses, or from a direct approach to the department by the person concerned. The potential client's need for care is then assessed. In some respects the home help's links with the informal network may be closer than those to other formal services. Pilot research in Dinnington by Bayley (1982, p. 194) showed that due to longer hours worked, geographical concentration of clients and local knowledge, home helps and wardens occupied a special position in the village and straddled the boundary between statutory services and informal care. The other professionals, however, did not exploit this knowledge, and there was little contact with social workers, health visitors and others. Dexter and Harbert's recent comprehensive discussion of the home help service (1983), apart from a token general discussion of informal care, says virtually nothing about the potential for using the service to link formal and informal care, suggesting that such overlap which does occur is not planned but is a function of the type of people who work as home helps and their local base.

Available resources determine the level of service provided. The number of home helps for every thousand elderly people varies widely between authorities. The national average is 6.8, but that conceals a wide variability – between Newcastle on Tyne with 16 per 1,000, Camden with 14, Sheffield with 12, through Gwent with 10, Lancashire with 6 to Powys with 4 and the Isle of Wight, Surrey and Kingston-on-Thames with 3. Some authorities provide the service free, others charge (with some of the users being assessed on their income). Such crude comparisons reflect the age structure of the authorities, not their socioeconomic structure or the extent of deprivation among the elderly. But they undoubtedly conceal differing philosophies of home help provision, with an inclination to higher expenditure on the part of Labour authorities (Sharpe and Newton, 1984; Phyllis Willmott, 1984).

In the debate about formal and informal care, some advocates of the free market place a good deal of emphasis upon non-statutory sources of care. Other observers point to social changes which affect informal care and the certainty provided by statutory provision, since only government has the resources and authority to plan effectively (Graycar, 1983, p. 391).

BALANCE THEORY

Practice, then, is variable, as is the extent of interpenetration of formal and informal care. Certainly, interweaving has a considerable appeal to policy-makers as a future goal. The extent to which it can be realized, however, depends on the ways in which formal and informal care can fit together, as well as on what is attempted in the way of practical solutions. This needs to be considered conceptually, for there may be logical obstacles to interweaving to which insufficient attention has been given by its advocates.

The most optimistic view of statutory and informal care has been formulated in abstract terms by Litwak and Meyer (1966), who set out a balance theory of co-ordination between bureaucratic organizations and primary groups in the locality. They observe that social scientists have tended to focus upon two polar opposites, the Weberian ideal type of bureaucracy on the one hand, and the warmth and intimacy of the family on the other. This antithesis has been exaggerated, and both types of care are essential for achieving most social tasks. However, the right balance must be struck. If the bureaucratic organization and external primary group are too isolated from each other they are likely to interfere with one another and reduce their contributions to achieving a goal. If they are brought too close together, however, their antithetical atmospheres are likely to disrupt one or both organizations.

> Optimum social control is likely to occur when coordinating mechanisms develop between bureaucratic organisations and external primary groups that balance their relationships at a midpoint of social distance where they are not too intimate and not isolated from each other. This formulation requires recognition of the importance of a variety of mechanisms of coordination, ranging from those capable of bridging great social distances to those capable of increasing distance, while maintaining communication (Litwak and Meyer, 1966, p. 38)

Applied to formal and informal care, the idea is that where formal and informal care are not too intimate and not too isolated from one another, an optimum balance is achieved. A key element in this is the notion of linkage, and the idea that linkages may be fostered where the two are too remote or may be reduced where the two are too close (Litwak, 1985, p. 27; see also, Litwak, Meyer and Hollister, 1977 for its application to education and health).

The concept is stimulating in that it goes beyond strict organization theory to look at the connections between organizations and their external environment. However, its formulation of the relations between the two types of care is too bland, and its postulation of 'balance' begs a whole series of questions, both about the relative power and influence of each and of the extent to which each 'matches' the other. These weaknesses derive from an underlying functionalism that postulates that there are certain societal goals which are met by bureaucratic organizations and others which are met by community primary groups. This, however, is highly questionable, and moreover throws little light upon how formal and informal care may interact. The two types of care need not necessarily be 'balanced' – one may predominate – neither are they necessarily complementary in the way that 'balance' theory implies.

Another related approach, adopted by Marvin Sussman (1977) has been to look at the linkage groups by which relations between primary groups and bureaucracies are effected, mediated or constrained. He identifies five: kinship networks, peer groups, special interest groups, voluntary associations and ombudsman systems. He discusses how care is provided for the dependent elderly, and envisages various ways in which those people and their close associates may deal with bureaucracy. Individual family members can clearly play a major role. Friends drawn from the peer group can do so in some circumstances. Membership of a self-help group may be a source of linkage in other circumstances. The reference to ombudsman systems envisages the possibility of someone acting as an advocate on a person's behalf. Sussman is less sanguine than Litwak and Meyer, observing that bureaucracy has usually been in a superordinate position and the family in a subordinate position viewed as a whole. Is it possible, he asks, to have co-ordination rather than conflict between bureaucratic organizations and primary groups?

DISCONTINUITIES BETWEEN FORMAL AND INFORMAL CARE

Less optimistic but more fruitful formulations have been proposed by Philip Abrams (1984) and Charles Froland (1980), both more impressed by the possible discontinuities between formal and informal care and critical of the idea of a continuum of care. The discussion which follows draws upon their ideas, also emphasizing that a single principle such as 'balance' is inadequate. Different types of relationship are possible, and all situations cannot be combined into a single model.

Colonization

The first and perhaps dominant relationship between formal and informal care can be a colonization by the formal of the informal. The informal sector and the locality are invaded by statutory and voluntary services and subordinated to their ends. Characteristically orientated both to service delivery of care and to control, their common strategy is to create dependency. Typically, the formal provision of services is substituting for the efforts of the informal network. Such substitute care from formal services cannot normally provide the person cared for with enough dignity, self esteem and active membership in local networks for satisfactory survival (Barker, 1980, p. 159). So he or she becomes dependent and in some situations passive. (Even though this discussion focuses upon the form of the organization of care, these effects on the cared for must not be lost sight of.)

Domination is the most explicit form of colonization. Here, statutory or voluntary agencies merely impose their own preferred forms of bureaucratic control over informal systems. Holmes and Maizels's study of social workers and volunteers (1979), for example, shows how social workers excluded volunteers from all kinds of case work and limited their role of 'befriending' to doing practical tasks for the elderly and physically handicapped, and generally working with client groups social workers themselves were least involved with. Roles are ordered to fit the categories of the organization, and informal carers are given subordinate responsibilities at a low level.

Appropriation is a somewhat less explicit form of colonization. Boundaries are again drawn, but in such a way as to redefine the limits of the formal and informal sectors, usually including what had been informal in an expanded definition of the formal. A good example is provided by the movement to register childminders. Attempts to co-ordinate informal with formal care may involve transferring informal gate-keepers or 'central figures' (Collins and Pancoast, 1976) into the formal system, thus tidying things up bureaucratically at the expense of the open-endedness, unconventionality and loose ends of informal provision.

Co-option is an attempt to foster local participation in larger organizations, which involves the formal sphere trying to build some element of informality into its own approach. For example, attempts to use 'indigenous paraprofessionals' as bridges to poor areas in American cities show some tendency for these informal helpers to take on professional roles and come to identify more with the interests of the formal organization (Froland, 1980, p. 578). Informal local information and intelligence systems have been turned into resources within the formal sector to enable services to be delivered more effectively to those in need. Colonization was involved, however, since the aim was to improve the delivery of formal care.

Abrams observes that the outcome under any of these three

forms is less due to power lust on the part of formal agencies as 'the hypnotic fascination of the powerful for the powerless (as in the early history of the British Empire) . . . Formalization is the order of the day – preferably through rather loose and discrete links, but nevertheless the problem is to get organized: rather a well-run colony than a mere tribe' (Abrams, 1984, p. 425).

Competition or conflict?

Not all denizens of the informal sector, however, steer this course, and an alternative mode of interaction may be competition or conflict between two sectors. Competition occurs when there is a common perception of need but ambivalence in the assessments of responsibility or the capacity of available alternatives for providing care. Residential care for the elderly is currently one field in Britain where there is competition between statutory and private market provision. Nursery education is another, although statutory provision in this area has been minimal. Competition is a way of providing alternative options for care which can often be fostered by a minimalist policy of government provision, leaving the way open for other forms of care.

Conflict arises where those involved in informal networks are at odds with policies for care being pursued by government. Classic examples are provided by the welfare rights movement in Britain (Rose, 1974) and the civil rights movement in the United States. Both sought to bring pressure on government to change both the substance of policies and the way in which those policies were administered. Of perhaps greater interest have been those groups, arising from shared individual experience of informal care, which have sought to articulate the demands of those cared for and bring pressure to bear on government for policy change (cf. Richardson and Goodman, 1983). Examples in Britain include MENCAP (for the mentally handicapped), Disabled Drivers, Gingerbread (for single parents) and the Patients' Association. In some cases their main role is to act as self-help groups, but one of their principal characteristics is that of translating need into demand, articulated as a pressure group through the political system, rather than accepting of care. As in the different case of local residents' groups concerned with planning issues, such activities 'demonstrate the possibility of intensifying the soli-darity and effectiveness of informal neighbourhood networks through conflict' (Abrams, 1984, p. 426). Unlike planning action groups, however, which tend to be neighbourhood-based, action groups for care are more likely to be formed on the basis of 'shared fate' (being dependent upon public assistance, having a mentally handicapped child, etc) and are not confined to the immediate locality. The implications of this will be examined further below. The notion of a continuum of care fails adequately to recognize that conflict may be built into relations between the formal and the informal. For

> 'the *objectives* of informal welfare may on occasion be rather different from those of formal services. . . . If social workers are to 'tap' the informal, they need to be alert to the very real possibility of deep-seated conflicts. . . . Studies of informal welfare should not forestall or distort the process of recognis-ing such conflicts by making assumptions about the univer-sality of certain meanings. Too often this is inadequately grasped' (Offer, 1984, p. 552).

A further aspect to be attended to is the possibility of compe-tition, cleavage and conflict within each of the two types of care, the formal and informal sectors. It is a mistake to treat them as monoliths. In Britain, for example, there is a clear division of responsibility between local authority social services and the health services. Despite some nominal mechanisms for co-ordination, in practice, to a very large extent, both go their own way and pursue policies independently. Though in most respects their activities are complementary, this can lead to con-flict or competition in some circumstances. For example, it is proving difficult to share responsibility for the discharged inmates of mental handicap and mental illness hospitals because the purse-strings are controlled by health authorities, and local authority social service and housing departments are unwilling to take on additional responsibilities without the resources to fund them. In the informal sector, there has generally been insufficient attention to the possibilities of cleavage at the local level in mobilizing informal networks. Two types rather obviously come to mind. One is the conflicting interests at the very local, street, level between elderly people and families with young children over children's play activities, which interfere with the peace and quiet of the area. (For one example see Bulmer, 1986a, pp. 80–1).

A different type of cleavage may run along ethnic lines. As many parts of British inner cities are now multi-ethnic in character this is an important consideration. A degree of social distance characterizes relations between different ethnic groups, and informal ties tend to be within each group. This is particularly marked among those coming from the Indian sub-continent. Abrams and his team describe a neighbourhood care scheme in a Midlands town in a racially mixed area, one of whose achievements was to break down racial barriers and get local whites and Asians to know each other a bit better (Bulmer, 1986a, p. 149; Abrams et al., 1986, pp. 64–80). The significance of ethnic attachment in discussions of informal care has not had enough attention (for a recent exception see Thomas, 1986). As Gerald Suttles has observed (1968), residents of inner city areas search for trustworthy associates in a population where the grounds of trustworthiness tend to be scarce. In the absence of any other basis for trust, ethnic ties are a primordial attachment that people tend to fall back upon. Other cleavages may exist along gender or social class lines at the local level.

Coexistence

Colonization represents the pull of the formal sector, competition or conflict a mutual challenge from differing standpoints. Coexistence represents a degree of mutual insulation of each sphere from the other. According to Froland, this is the most popular or characteristic relationship between the formal and informal sectors (Froland, 1980, p. 578). The lack of interaction may stem from ignorance, indifference, mutual disregard or a judgement that there are no relevant grounds for interaction. In some cases, helping patterns are known to occur within families or among neighbours and friends, but the care involved is too spontaneous to be taken account of by formal efforts. In other cases the link has been disavowed, as in the case of mutual aid and self-help groups who do not want formal involvement, but are not in a relationship of conflict with the formal sector. There is little motivation on either side to try to link the two sides, so they coexist without interacting. The same is true of informal caring efforts that are outside the limits of public policy concerns, but are of live importance to those involved in informal activity. Examples of these would be women's groups at a local level, gay and lesbian networks, and other consciousness-raising or self-improvement activities. Certain British local authorities have provided funding for women's rights and gay rights, which may tend toward colonization. The general rule, however, is that these are not seen as proper concerns for the formal sector and so the informal activity coexists alongside, and is insulated from, the formal sector, without conflict between the two.

Collaboration

If colonization, conflict and coexistence are three modes which keep formal and informal care from making a complementary contribution, collaboration between the two, the mode which underpins the model of 'interweaving', also occurs. Froland observes that:

> the best examples of collaboration seem to arise on an *ad hoc* basis, as when a professional is able to form a consultative relationship with a neighbourhood helper who provides friendly reassurance to elderly neighbours; an outreach team is able to form an informal support system of hotel managers, board and care operators, bartenders and grocery clerks in promoting the community adjustment of the chronically mentally ill; or when informal working relationships are established between mutual aid or self-help groups and professionals (Froland, 1980, p. 579).

The difficulties of sustaining such collaboration are considerable. There are numbers of pressures (considered below) which push care either in the formal or the informal direction. Even Bayley, a sympathetic advocate, recognizes 'the danger of the formal system taking over and/or destroying the informal system' (Bayley, 1982, p. 185). What is required is a sufficient strengthening of the informal sector to enable it to deal on equal terms with the formal sector and avoid the fate of incorporation. The values and relationships of the informal sector need to be respected and sustained. Statutory and voluntary agencies would have to learn to live with the informal sector as an equal.

There is also a clear political dimension to genuine collaboration. 'Whether or not one goes as far as some American city governments, some serious surrender of powers is unavoidable if one really wants any significant measure of social care to be provided within neighbourhood social networks' (Abrams, 1980, p. 23). It is this requirement for give-and-take which makes it so difficult to achieve collaboration in practice. Because of their responsibility and accountability within a bureaucratic organization, formal care-givers tend to push toward the colonization mode, whether they intend to or not. This is why, over time, collaboration tends to move toward other modes of collaboration.

Confusion

A final mode of relationship between formal and informal care is confusion. There is a tension between the resources available through the formal system and the values of the informal system. Those involved are unsure how to resolve this tension. Should one try to retain the element of informality, even at the expense of satisfying the conditions required for formal support? Or should one accept formal support and run the risk of professionalizing what is essentially an informal relationship? The issue of payment to volunteers, discussed below, is a good example of the type of issues at the boundaries of formal and informal care which can easily lead to confusion. This mode of interaction is of more than passing importance, since a good deal of government policy in this area might fairly be characterized as either based on, or likely to lead to, confusion. The failure to think through what 'community care' involves, and its continued use as a rhetorical device in discussions of care policy, contributes materially to confusion.

OBSTACLES TO INTERWEAVING.

The notion of a continuum of care, or of 'interweaving', is thus considerably more difficult to implement than appears at first sight. Care *in* the community is difficult to convert into care *by* the community, particularly if this means having formal and informal carers working in close co-operation with each other.

The ideal and the reality are quite far apart. It is all very well to identify the different modes the relationship may fall into, but what accounts for these different outcomes? An attempt will now be made to identify some of the factors which inhibit the interweaving of formal and informal care, before considering ways in which the two might be brought closer together.

Client Autonomy

One of the characteristics or informal care is its capacity to sustain the person cared for as an autonomous and self-respecting individual. Such care enables individuals to exist as normal adults, with minimal interference from outsiders, retaining their independence and, within physical limits, freedom of movement. To be sure this is not true of all dependants. The mentally handicapped child or adult, or the dementing elderly person, for instance, may not be capable of such self-determination. It is, however, true of the majority of the elderly and the physically handicapped that they are capable of such autonomy. Thus, formal services which support that autonomy are appreciated and used. Writing of the elderly, Jonathan Barker observes that:

> people stress the value of such things as chiropody, denture repair services, opticians, unobtrusive hearing aids, bus passes and advice services. Also highly appreciated are the services of most home helps who have the capacity to enable a person to keep her home in a state of which, as she is accustomed, she can be proud enough to invite in neighbours and grandchildren (Barker, 1980, p. 168).

Such 'enabling' help is distinguished from help which elderly people and their relatives and friends see as 'disabling'. A prime example is resistance to suggestions to accept a place in residential care, since it involves accepting not only that the individual concerned is no longer independent but that he or she may be treated objectively, as a person not fully able to cope, by staff in the institutional setting.

In a recent study of the elderly in rural north Wales, Clare Wenger places a similar emphasis upon the need for a collaborative approach to problem solving involving elderly people, their close relatives, and significant others in their personal network.

The role of the helping professional could encourage the individual and the family or other potential carers to look at options, perhaps hitherto unconsidered. Such an approach would, of course, necessitate a change in perspectives. It becomes necessary to see the old person in most cases as potentially competent and as active in decisions about his or her future rather than as the passive recipient of resources. . . . The data suggest that the majority are able and willing to solve their own problems but that they may need support to do this. (Wenger, 1984, p. 189)

A recognition of the value in fostering independence is a very important strength of informal ties, and this is perhaps the most important point to be recognized in seeking to link informal and formal care. The elderly, for example, may fight shy of having a social worker because it marks them off, in their own eyes and those of others, as 'needing help', and having their autonomy or dignity infringed. Moreover, it involves identification with other social work clients, such as 'problem families', with whom association is a stigma. One advantage of district nurses as workers from the formal sector contributing to the care of the elderly is that they are less likely to be seen as providing a 'disabling' service.

The Role of Local Authorities

Mention of the aims and objectives of social work leads on to a second point about informal and formal care, the objectives which are being pursued in providing care. Lack of clarity about this has undoubtedly led to confusion when attempts have been made to interweave the two types of care. This particularly applies to the activities of local authority Social Services departments. A distinction may be made between three types of activity that they undertake. First, social workers help individuals and families to maintain and develop their capacities by counselling. Secondly, specialist services provide activities such as occupational therapy, education and training for groups like children and the handicapped, and mobility aids. Thirdly, services are directed to meeting basic human needs such as feeding, clothing and cleanliness, many of which may be met by informal carers but which Social Services may meet in some circumstances (Dexter and Harbert, 1983, pp. 172–3). The prevailing image of Social Services departments as mainly delivering social work is thus rather misleading. In the field of care, home help services, meeting the third set of needs, are arguably more important. The Barclay Report explicitly recognized that a redefinition of the role of the social worker was required, by means of a shift from a concern with counselling to one with social care planning. Where it lay itself open to criticism was in failing to specify how social care planning was to be organized and focused, given the multiple objectives pursued by Social Services departments.

The Geography of Care

A third critical area in which there has been lack of clarity has been the geographical area at which particular types of provision are targeted. This applies both to the organization of formal care and to assumptions which are made about the existence of informal care. In considering care in any urban area, four levels of geographical aggregation can usefully be distinguished. These are as follows.

(1)   *The street.* This is a group of contiguous dwellings which form a unit. They may extend upwards as a tower block, as well as lengthwise as a street, but they are the primary reference point for local residents once they go beyond their own house. The numbers involved will vary, as residents draw boundaries in different ways (for example, in very long streets), but the mode would be about 100 residents.

(2)   *The 'village'.* The reference here is to a larger unit comprising a number of streets, such as a rural village or an urban 'village' of a traditional kind such as Roberts (1971) described for Salford, or the basic unit within a new town (like Washington in County Durham) laid out on a dispersed pattern. The American term 'neighbourhood' is an alternative. The upper limit of the number of residents in such an area would be about 5,000, but it could be smaller. It would be small enough for all the young children to go to the same primary school. This unit also corresponds to what Janowitz and Suttles call the 'social bloc', which arises primarily from the indigenous processes associated with the locality, resulting from propinquity, homogeneity, natural boundaries and a

diffuse pattern of interaction, and tending to homogeneity (Janowitz and Suttles, 1978, pp. 96–7).

(3) *The district.* This refers to a subdivision of a town or city which contains a number of villages or neighbourhoods, which together constitute a recognizable part of a larger whole. Areas such as Tufnell Park or Highgate in London, Fenham or Byker in Newcastle-on-Tyne, Hyde Park or the Near North Side in Chicago are examples of districts. A district also corresponds roughly to what in Chicago urban sociology was called a 'natural area' (Hunter, 1974). Its population is variable, but the mode is about 30,000 residents, very considerably larger than a neighbourhood. Small towns with a population below 50,000 may be regarded as districts, composed of villages and streets – that is, they can be considered at just three levels of aggregation. Districts will tend to be larger in a city than in a medium-sized town.

(4) *The town.* Above the district lies the town, a larger unit made up of several districts with a population in excess of 100,000. Many towns are identifiable urban areas with clear boundaries. Within large cities, however, the term may be used to refer to *sections* of the city (such as the East End of London, or the South Side of Chicago) or to *administrative units,* such as the London Borough of Haringey or the Borough of Queens in New York.

(5) *The city.* In large conurbations, the city is the largest unit, with a population of, or exceeding, 1 million.

In providing care, interest focuses upon the smaller units; the fifth, the city, will be disregarded for the purposes of the present discussion.

Table 6.1 shows types of both formal and informal care provided at different levels within a typical British urban area. Discussions of the complementarity of informal and formal care have usually by-passed any distinctions in terms of area level, and so have missed important points about the possibilities for substituting or 'interweaving' care (for one exception see Hunter and Riger, 1986, pp. 68–9). For example, if it is proposed that the district nurse or social worker co-ordinates care with neighbours of the person cared for, not only is the relationship to the cared for person very different, but the geographical basis is quite different. The social worker is not familiar with the local milieu, does not

Table 6.1   *Types of Informal and Formal Care Provided at Different Area Levels within a Typical British Urban Area*

	Informal	Formal
Street	Next-door-neighbours Other neighbours	
Village or neighbourhood	Local social network, dependent on (a) length of local residence (b) age and stage of life cycle (c) number of local relatives	Home help service Home/street wardens
District	'Good neighbour' and neighbourhood care schemes	District/community nurse Social work area team
Town	Self-help groups (e.g. Gingerbread, AA) Friends Relatives	Specialist social services provision Community psychiatric nurse Residential care Geriatric hospital care

interact with local people on a day-to-day basis, and will necessary at first be seen as an outsider and therefore more distant. Similarly, specialist social service provision from the town level has an even greater gap to cross if it seeks to link to informal care provided at street or village level. On the informal side, many neighbourhood care schemes (such as those described by Abrams and his team (1986)) are not specifically local either, but extend across at least a district area. As explained in Chapter 2, informal networks are by no means purely confined to the street or village level, whether with relatives, friends or activities within self-help organizations. So there is a much greater mix both on the formal and informal side, and meshing care involves taking account of these levels as well as other conditions which are conducive to success.

Locally-Based Services

So far as the organization of formal services is concerned, some observers have argued that a shift to 'interweaving' must be accompanied by moves to decentralize authority and provide locally based services. Decentralization involves delegating power to allocate resources down to a more local level than the city, town or district. The Kent Community Care scheme (Challis and Davies, 1980) was one experimental project to give local Social Services managers freedom to work within a given budget, and to use part of that budget to pay informal carers to work under the umbrella of the local Social Services department. The idea of community empowerment in America reflects the move to decentralization, but this has not been taken up to any extent in Britain. What has been pursued by a few local authorities are plans to decentralize and reorganize services so that they are delivered at a neighbourhood level from offices staffed by social workers, housing officials and environmental health officers, under a local manager. Islington, for example, is one London borough which is following this path. Potentially, such decentralization offers considerable scope for meshing with local informal networks. Whether this can in fact be done remains to be seen. Some other obstacles, discussed below, may militate against this happening.

The idea of providing services locally does not necessarily entail the idea of decentralizing authority, although it may do. The most striking example in Britain is provided by those local authorities which have created a 'patch'-based local system of social work, with social workers, rather than working from area teams, made individually responsible for small 'patches' of about 5,000–10,000 people (corresponding to the village) within which they are responsible for generic care (see Hadley and McGrath, 1984). The theory is that social workers will know their areas more intimately, and be better able to liaise with other services provided locally, such as home helps, as well as being able to mesh with the local informal networks. It is too early to reach a firm conclusion on the merits of 'patch' and it is the subject of heated professional debate. But some pointers to the problems involved are provided in Bayley *et al*'s. (1984) study of Dinnington. He found that in a locally co-ordinated office, while social workers, housing officials and health staff worked effectively together, it was more difficult to liaise effectively with the home help services, who, in turn, did not seem to be particularly effective in integrating their services with the informal support from kin and neighbours which their clients received. It is unwise to generalize from this case, but it is clear that local provision of services *in themselves* is not a panacea if other problems are ignored.

A more radical approach is needed to formal service delivery if interweaving is to be made to work. Clare Wenger, on the basis of her Welsh research, sketches out what this might be.

Interweaving is *not* about shifting responsibility from statutory services on to informal providers. Neither is it about co-opting and colonising informal systems or about superimposing existing packages of care on the community. If interweaving is to work well, it must start from the perspective of the community or the locality as a caregiving system by seeking to reinforce and optimise existing resources and creating resources to fill gaps in provision. It therefore requires familiarity with family and neighbourhood networks; consultation with network members as well as clients, development of partnerships with other social services, such as doctors' practices, schools, churches and voluntary organisations; and . . . a requirement to view the whole community as both needing and offering support (Wenger, 1983, p. 48).

Organizational Constraints

At this point, one begins to run up against some of the obstacles hinted at earlier which are inherent in working within formal organizations. Colonization occurs for reasons to do with roles, skills, responsibilities and accountability of those who work within the formal sector. The theory of interweaving is that professionals can handle problems requiring technical expertise, special knowledge and detachment, while informal carers cope with problems of a long-term nature requiring emotional support. Such a partnership is not easy to accomplish in practice. First, formal and informal carers differ in the time commitment which they bring to care. Being employed to provide care establishes certain expectations, including the notion of fixed duration – hours of work or a shift – while informal care, particularly in the family, has no beginning and end unless relief care is available. Roles of professionals and those of informal care-givers are different. It cannot be assumed that the two will easily co-exist. For example, in the care of mentally handicapped children, the demands made on parents are very onerous and without respite. Bayley's study of such families (1973) showed that short visits from social workers intended to provide emotional support were of little help to the parents. What would have been of much more use, but was not available, was respite care. Lack of complementarity was due in part to the different time frames of the informal and formal carers. The one was open-ended and limitless, the other fixed and short-term as part of working day covering many cases.

A second respect in which the formal and informal carer is different lies in the knowledge which each brings to bear on the caring task. Professionals are trained in technical skills of various kinds, and possess specialized information. Whether social workers or occupational therapists or district nurses, they have been trained to deal with specific aspects of the human condition. Informal carers, on the other hand, base their actions on personal knowledge, whether acquired through experience, background or culture. It has been argued, for example, that women tend to adopt caring roles in part because of the nurturant role which they play as mothers, and which they observe in their own mothers (Gilligan, 1982; Noddings, 1984). Informal carers form ties that are particularistic and ascriptive, whereas formal carers are thoroughly imbued with an orientation to rational action. 'The references for professionals are formal training, other professionals, career aspirations and the immediate working environment, while references for the informal helper centre on shared needs, experiences and traditions within a set of relationships with others' (Froland, 1980, p. 580). Professionals may, for example, lack the skills necessary to promote interweaving. One aspect of informal care is the stress that builds up for carers. A study by Sainsbury and De Alarçon (1974) showed that visiting psychiatrists were better at detecting demented or antisocial elderly people than they were at identifying those with neurotic tendencies or personality disorders who could be just as wearing on their families.

A consequence of superior knowledge is not infrequently status differences which hinder collaboration. The expertise of the professional or bureaucrat often translates into a judgement of superior knowledge. Problems and solutions come increasingly to be defined in terms drawn from formal care. Informal care-givers are seen as needing training to acquire some degree of professional skill. As a result, supervision of informal by formal care-givers results, instead of collaboration. The perspectives of the informal care given, or the ways in which the informal sector can handle problems, are ignored or devalued. It is instructive that one of the more effective forms of formal care – the home help service – is one where status differences between carer and cared for are minimized. There may well be a connection between this and the one-fifth of home helps who say they are doing neighbourly acts for their clients in their own time (Goldberg and Connelly, 1982, p. 169).

Accountability

The dilemma of accountability poses one of the most formidable obstacles to interweaving different types of care. Social Services staff are part of a local government structure in which they are subordinate to managers who themselves are answerable to the chief executive and committees of elected representatives. Though in practice they have quite high degrees of professional autonomy, the need for accountability represents a major obstacle to experiments with money or people. It is noteworthy that attempts at interweaving have been attempted much more with the elderly, where social workers are little involved, than with children, where they have tightly-drawn statutory responsibilities. Informal involvement in child care is confined to managing parental contact (for children in care), fostering on a paid basis, or adoption, whereby responsibility is completely transferred by law to the new parents.

At one level this involves money. 'Accountants demand financial returns that stretch beyond what is reasonable for the recording capacities of front-line staff and informal carers; managers, at the behest of committees, demand referral back of decisions which, if not made rapidly while informal carers are motivated, may never be implemented (Darvill, 1983, p. 256). But it is also a matter of attitude of mind. Working within large formal organizations does not encourage the flexibility and speed of reaction needed to maximize the contribution of informal carers to joint care. One virtue of experiments such as the Kent Community Care Scheme is that they encourage not only new organizational forms but also place staff in a position where they have to radically re-think their responsibilities.

Accountability is not just a problem between the formal and informal sectors. It is also a problem within different parts of the formal sector. Problems of accountability arise in the health services as well as personal social services, and, if anything, hierarchical thinking and deference to lines of authority are even stronger in these areas. The perennial problems arising from trying to encourage liaison between health services and personal social services derive to a considerable extent from these factors. Even within particular services, line accountability may hinder co-operation with other groups. (Problems of co-ordination between the home help service and other parts of Social Services departments have already been mentioned.)

Whatever the rhetorical allegiance to crossing lines of administrative authority, in practice it is extraordinarily difficult to achieve successfully. An experienced North American observer of the phenomenon, Alexander Leighton, a social psychiatrist, writes:

> Interagency cooperation is generally even more troublesome than intra-agency cooperation. Any real change in relations between agencies will require drastic alterations in the shared sentiments within the civil service and also within the professions. One influence of importance could be mobilised if administrators were to act so as to make cooperation rewarding. As things are, despite universal praise of cooperation, there is almost no encouragement for carrying it out. For some years I have made it a practice to ask administrators at all levels in hospitals, outpatient services, social agencies and other related types of institutions the following question: 'When was the last time you promoted someone for interagency cooperation?' The answer is almost always a surprised look, an awkward

silence, and then some version of 'If I am honest, I'll have to say "never" '. (Leighton, 1982, pp. 217–8)

Accountability, then, raises formidable difficulties. Proponents of interweaving, on the other hand, have generally failed to think through the problem of accountability and to suggest ways in which new lines of responsibility can be established to make care a genuinely collaborative activity.

Emotional Content and Loading

One major dimension of difference between the two types of care lies in the emotional content and loading, which differ between formal and informal carers. The former tend to be emotionally detached, the latter more involved – though with negative as well as positive feelings expressed. Thus, difference in the emotional content and loading of care has an important bearing on the potential for collaboration.

> 'Sharing' care has an attractive sound to it, it is commendable. That does not mean to say that it is easily realised. It may be hard to achieve emotionally and, practically, it may be exceedingly complicated to organise. We know, for instance, how difficult it is for the parent of the child in care to share that child's care in any meaningful fashion with residential care staff or with foster parents. Sharing care may mean sharing love or sharing anguish and pain. Not least, adults who have experienced independence may be reluctant to share their self-care with others. In fact, if one looks carefully at how tending is organised, the succession of responsibility is much more common than genuine sharing. (Parker, 1981, p. 24)

The example given earlier of the elderly person (p. 176) makes the point about succession of responsibility very clearly.

Within the informal sphere, 'sharing care' may also be problematical. The most striking examples of successful sharing are provided by care between spouses. With this exception, gender remains a powerful obstacle to sharing care. The great bulk of those who look after the dependent elderly, the long-term sick, the handicapped and young children, are women. In the formal sector also, women predominate as carers, especially among home helps and the staffs of residential and children's homes. A good deal of attention has been paid to such biases in care (for example, Finch and Groves, 1980; Finch and Groves, 1983; Ungerson, 1987). The biases remain entrenched and place limits on the extent to which 'sharing care' can be pursued.

Different ideological outlooks influence the efficacy of 'interweaving'. One has heard a good deal of the virtues of collaboration in the formal sector in recent years. Too little attention has been paid to the recipients of care. They and their relatives and friends may hold values which make the acceptance of formal care difficult, just as receipt of non-contributory state income support arouses feelings of stigma and state charity.

Political and Ethical Considerations

Political interests are also involved in interweaving. To the extent that particular political parties become proponents of interweaving, collaborative care can become a political background. Currently, much emphasis is placed by the Conservative government upon the virtues of voluntary effort and self-help, but it is not clear how far these are meant to extend. Evidence was quoted earlier (see p. 180) showing that home help services were more extensive in Labour-controlled local authorities. Consistent policies for collaboration are too new to be able to judge how difficult they may be to implement but undoubtedly difficulties could arise in the future.

Finally, a constellation of issues – part political, part ethical, part sociological – concern the extent of intrusiveness of the formal sector and what the 'social care planning' advocated by the Barclay Report might actually mean in practice. For collaborative care implies that formal carers will be more or less well informed about the needs of potential clients, and will seek to intervene to mobilize the most effective package of care possible. This is already happening for elderly people or the mentally disturbed on discharge from hospital, and in the field of mental health the 'key worker' with overall responsibility for an ex-patient has assumed some importance. But how far can such an approach be applied to other types of dependency, and how far can it be extended to embrace, for example, relative strangers in the neighbourhood.

Professional workers have their own ethical codes and norms, but these are often narrowly applied within one field of professional practice (such as medicine) and may hinder inter-professional communication because other groups (such as social workers) are considered less responsible in ethical terms. At best, information may be shared on a 'need-to-know' basis between fellow professionals concerned with particular clients. Entirely new problems are created, however, when it is proposed to share information about a client with a neighbourhood care-giver who is part of that person's informal network. Some of these privacy implications were considered more fully in Chapter 3 (see also, Bulmer, 1987). The point was made polemically by Robert Pinker in his dissent to Barclay (1982, p. 256) when he referred to 'today's secular welfare evangelicals, who wish to advertise their services in every pub, pulpit and private residence in the country'.

Preventative social care is also a political issue. It can be argued that the state should not be permitted to intrude too far into the private, informal worlds of kin, neighbours and friends. Is it acceptable, as Pinker puts it, to license strangers, including volunteers, to inquire into the personal circumstances of citizens who have neither asked for help nor committed any offence? Will interweaving, Giles Darvill asked,

> provide the different forms of the public world, including neighbourhood groups, with channels for spreading their tentacles into the privacy of family life further than is acceptable? Will we be forced to be active, forbidden to be lazy? Will grandma and her granddaughter ever be allowed to be free of each other? (Darvill, 1983, p. 258)

Sociological issues of privatization also bear on the matter. 'No one else could cope with my mother' is a familiar phrase to would-be volunteers, but the sociological foundations of such suspicion and the tendency to privatize family problems are poorly understood. Does inadequacy seek to hide its head rather than share the anguish and pain? Outsiders offering care and support *may* be welcomed, but they may not, and the underlying trend toward more dispersed networks and a degree of withdrawal into the nuclear family, discussed in Chapter 2, certainly suggests that if such help is offered from a local source, it may not be welcomed without considerable reservations.

FOSTERING INTERWEAVING MORE REALISTICALLY

The discussion of the obstacles to interweaving formal and informal care is by no means intended to suggest that the two are not capable of being linked, rather that the obstacles to their linkage have tended to be lost sight of in academic and political enthusiasm for the policy. Nor is the discussion intended to overlook the social factors encouraging the growth of collaboration between formal and informal sectors. Social trends indicating greater need and demand – particularly the growing number of elderly people over the age of 75 – have highlighted the importance of extending the boundaries of care. Criticism of the quality of care in formal institutions such as hospitals, residential homes and homes for the mentally handicapped, has led both to decarceration and the aim of keeping people in their own homes for as long as possible. Cutbacks in public spending make various forms of 'community' care appear cheaper alternatives (whether in reality they are cheaper is another matter). In some quarters there has been a strong desire to combine the best of statutory provision with local community mobilization. Advocates of decentralization of formal services have also seen such policies as being complementary to greater informal collaboration in care.

'Interweaving' remains an admirable aspiration, but from the point of view of policy, more thought needs to be given to the ways it can be fostered. One useful way of focusing the discussion is in terms of mediating structures, to ask what conditions need to be created so that informal and formal care can be brought together to flourish effectively. As background to this discussion, the necessity of formal, statutory services is assumed. As suggested earlier, informal care cannot by itself provide effective coverage of all needs. Though family care has great strengths, and plays a most active caring role, it has its limits. For government possesses a range of resources not available in informal care systems. Families cannot be expected to provide professional services in complex industrial societies (Graycar, 1983, p. 385).

Interwoven care is a mix of formal and informal care. One important practical question is: who copes in a crisis? For people with strong kin ties, relatives are likely to be the key figures, but for those without close kin, or with kin a long way away, formal carers may become more involved, particularly in situations such as discharge from hospital or bereavement for an elderly person. In this situation the formal role of 'key-worker' or 'care-co-ordinator' may be an appropriate one to establish. In practice, this role is sometimes taken on by hospital social workers (for example, in arranging hospital discharge) or by home help organizers. Too often, however, responsibility falls between different parts of the formal system. Different staff would be suitable to act as key-workers for clients loosely integrated into informal networks – it could be a social worker, or a district nurse, or a home help. The person filling such a role would liaise with the different formal services involved and with any informal carers involved, as well as consulting with the person being cared for.

The model for the 'key-worker' comes from the mental health field, with perhaps unfortunate overtones of a person unable to cope fully. A more appropriate parallel might be the local 'care manager' in schemes such as the Kent Community Care scheme, with responsibility and budget devolved to a local area office with the ability to 'buy-in' informal care. In other schemes involving 'patch' social work, the local social worker may play a key role in organizing the work of ancillary staff such as home helps from a local office, while at the same time trying to integrate voluntary and neighbourly efforts. In other models the district nurse could be the care co-ordinator. What all of these parallels suggest, however, is the importance of the need for sensitivity regarding the roles of informal carers, and the problem of how to effectively co-ordinate different formal services. Simply designating 'care-co-ordinators' will achieve nothing without structural changes which remove some of the obstacles to inter-organizational co-operation.

The 'key-worker' idea recognizes the importance which an individual can play in providing care. One study of the elderly, for example, showed that three-fifths of those receiving help obtained it from just one person, and only one in eight were helped by more than two people (Green, Creese and Kaufert, 1979). The aim of identifying central figures or 'sociometric stars' in the informal sector parallels the 'care-co-ordinator' approach in the formal sector. Central 'figures' in local informal networks are sought in a variety of roles such as local shopkeeper, publican, filling station attendant, crossing lady, milkman, and so on. They are seen as crucial gate-keepers between the formal and informal systems. Philip Abrams and his team describe a neighbourhood care scheme in an East Anglian town with an exceptionally vigorous local organizer, who treated it almost as a full-time job without payment. The scheme was entirely dependent upon her and was galvanized by her commitment. She was a 'central figure', without whom the scheme for visiting and befriending local people would have collapsed (Bulmer, 1986a, pp. 154–6; Abrams *et al.*, 1986, pp. 124–39).

Considerable weight in policy for informal caring is placed upon volunteers and the scope for expansion of such activity. Research on 'good neighbour' schemes suggests that a basic constraint is that the availability of volunteers is inversely proportional to the need of the area served, in other words, volunteers are more readily available in more prosperous middle-class areas, and in more affluent parts of the country, and less readily available in more working-class areas and poorer parts of the country (Abrams *et al.*, 1981, pp. 37–8). 'Suburban and rural areas with stable and affluent middle-class populations were more likely to generate voluntary action in 1980 than were urban areas with poor, ethnically mixed, working class and mobile populations' (K. Judge, quoted in Pinker, 1985, p. 110). Philip Abrams suggested that neighbourhood care schemes could be a basis for transforming neighbourly relations into friendship and a construct of actual or prospective exchange (Bulmer, 1986a, pp. 95–9). Specific schemes could become a vehicle for the fostering of friendship (rather than mere friendliness). The problem with neighbourhood care schemes would seem to be the unevenness of provision between and within areas, which makes purely voluntary effort by 'caring strangers' an uncertain means of promoting 'interweaving' of formal and informal care.

What has more potential would seem to be schemes which build upon mutual aid and self-help groups, where those who help are close to, or in the same position as, those being helped. A prime example of this is the care of the dependent elderly, in which the 'young old' (under 75) play an active part in a number of voluntary and statutory schemes around the country. There are also self-help groups such as the National Association of Widows, the National Council for the Single Woman and her Dependants, and Gingerbread, through which members get emotional support and advice and, in turn, pass it on to others (Richardson and Goodman, 1983). Care of mentally handicapped children devolves primarily upon the nuclear family, even extended kin playing a relatively restricted part. Where they exist, self-help voluntary bodies, such as mothers of mentally-handicapped children, can take some of the load to provide respite care, to allow for holidays or the occasional evening out (Barker, 1980, p. 164).

If voluntary activities are to flourish and to complement and supplement statutory services, then a great deal more thought and experimentation will have to be devoted to working out patterns of fruitful relationships between statutory-organised voluntary and informal neighbourhood activities in different local circumstances. . . . Since common experience and the results of several studies suggest that people of similar background and habits of living get on better than those living in very different social circumstances, ways of drawing in more working class volunteers will have to be found (Goldberg and Connelly, 1982, p. 178).

The prime means of drawing in more working-class volunteers is to develop schemes of payment for volunteers and informal helpers of one sort and another. A major part of the explanation for lack of volunteering on the middle-class pattern in working-class areas lies in the economic necessity of waged work to supplement the family income. Social policies which look upon volunteer effort as a free good by means of which informal care can substitute for statutory care are misleading and likely to lead to inadequate provision. Research by Qureshi, Challis and Davies (1983) showed that the prospect of financial reward was a motivating factor for as many as one-third of the volunteers which they studied. As Pinker convincingly suggests, 'one way of extending and strengthening supportive caring networks is to treat altruistic and pecuniary motives as complementary rather than antagonistic factors' (Pinker, 1985, p. 109).

Financial costs of providing informal care may vary. At one extreme, statutory bodies can meet the expenses of those running the scheme – for petrol and administrative expenses. Even here, quite high levels of subsidy may be provided, as, for example, hospitals which rely upon volunteer drivers to collect and deliver patients and pay them standard mileage allowances which involve quite large payments. A number of schemes, such as the Kent Community Care experiment, have tried paying participants in informal care schemes a nominal amount, of a few pounds a week, in recognition of the work that they are doing. At the other extreme, informal carers may be recruited and paid as waged workers, the prime example of this being the extension of the home help service by the appointment of local people as 'street wardens' to be involved in visiting the housebound and doing tasks such as shopping. Abrams and his team described one such scheme in a British northern industrial city, the participants in which were paid at home-help rates and were local authority employees (Bulmer, 1986a, pp. 122–6, 140–2).

The use of street wardens in a sense fused formal and informal care, since the wardens worked in the areas in which they lived, and might be known to the people they helped. More such arrangements need to be undertaken if the rhetoric of policy-makers about 'interweaving' is to be given any reality. These are difficult issues, of motivation, desert and comparability, in determining what level of payment is appropriate. Nominal payments may be criticized as demeaning, cheap labour and undercutting the rate for the job. Paying standard wages, on the other hand, might be regarded as undermining the voluntary principle, is very costly, and can, in certain circumstances, lead to colonization and displacement of objectives. Some method of payment, however, has already proved its worth in a number of schemes, particularly those involving working-class helpers, but more experimentation is needed to test the effects on recruitment and the impact on care of different forms of payment.

Encouraging complementarity between informal and formal care also involves more explicit attention to the family and resources within it. Reference has already been made to the withdrawal of home-help care if an elderly person has relatives who can help instead. Much more attention must be given to how the needs of various dependent groups can be encouraged through support for the family. This is a broad question to which feminist writers on social policy have paid particular attention, and the following are among the issues to be addressed. The underlying sociological issues concern the relative fixity or flexibility of men's and women's roles, and the extent to which caring tasks can be undertaken by men; and related to this, to what extent tending tasks may be undertaken by both sexes. At the policy level, fiscal policy toward family members who stay at home to look after kin needs reappraisal, since at present little support is available and existing benefits are meagre (Land, 1978). Means of enhancing family support by selective input of statutory services need refining, since too often it is assumed that, if the family is there, outside help is less necessary. In fact if the two are combined, the alternation of care such as is described in the case on p. 176 may be avoided. Care of the very dependent by family members is extremely stressful, and more attention is now focusing upon care for the carers, which may most effectively be provided from a statutory source or by fostering mutual aid groups (EOC, 1982; Briggs and Oliver, 1985).

Finally, the geographical and political framework within which services are provided will need adjustment if 'interweaving' of formal and informal care is to be realized on an extensive scale. Michael Bayley has put the general argument for services to be more locally based to promote interweaving.

A locally-based service makes it practicable and possible over time to become aware of and work with these local informal networks of care. . . . The local networks . . . include people other than just kith and kin. A locally based service makes it more practicable to establish contacts with other people who may be key figures in the network of support. They may be members of local voluntary organizations, shopkeepers, insurance men, the travelling shop. They may be other statutory workers such as staff of the local schools, doctors, the district nurse or the housing manager; they may be those most important workers who appear to play a key role in the relationship between the statutory and the informal sectors, that is home helps and wardens. It becomes possible to become involved in local issues which affect in a more general way the welfare of those in the area (Bayley, 1982, p. 186).

An interesting example of a proposal of this kind in an official report is the suggestion in the Cumberlege Report (DHSS, 1986, pp. 59–61) that health care associations should be created at the local level to represent consumer interests within the health service. These would be neighbourhood-level forums in which local people could contribute their views on health needs and health care planning, to influence decisions on the way services were provided by the new neighbourhood nursing service which Cumberlege recommended, and to complain if dissatisfied.

A negative example of how 'participation' may not work as intended is provided by a recent limited evaluation of 'patch' social work in East Sussex. Most respondents in the study know little about local social services and less about 'patch', even though it had been operating for some time.

> Whether as service users, workers or local residents, people's experience and views didn't seem to have made any impact on social services. None had ever been consulted over 'going local' and most felt they had little or no say in the department. 'Patch' had been much quicker to involve people in self-help than in self-management. Its rhetoric has been about participation, but its reality largely about organisational and management change (findings of Beresford and Croft, 1986, quoted by the authors in *The Guardian*, 25 June 1986).

This case, not necessarily generalizable, provides a vivid example of the gap between rhetoric and reality when it comes to interweaving, and shows how difficult it is to extend change within organizations to real changes in the way in which those organizations interact and deal with their external environment.

For such moves to be effective, they probably need to be linked to efforts to enhance local control, whereby non-institutional, small-scale and informal means of meeting people's needs can be found and exploited. In particular, means need to be worked out to enable effective representation at three of the levels discussed earlier, the neighbourhood, district and town levels (Table 6.1 – see p. 193). The issue is not the disappearance of the community on the one hand, or a simple juxtaposition between local and central control on the other. From the point of view of promoting 'interweaving', it is rather how formal and informal caring activities at the different levels can be intermeshed, and how the representational process can be modified to provide participation and accountability of those affected. This does not necessarily mean elected councils at each level. It does mean that much more serious attention should be paid at the village or district level to what Janowitz and Suttles (1978) call organizational communities, which may range from a very formal association to an informal group of concerned citizens.

Through organizational communities, citizens from the village or neighbourhood level can be involved in a wider, territorially based grouping, focused around the district level delivery of services. The need for such representation is underlined by the fact that, at the district level, responsibility is commonly divided between, for example, local authority social services, health services, local employment services, and voluntary organizations, with the problems of co-ordination and co-operation already discussed and often with a different geographical basis for each service. Organizational communities are not necessarily, or even usually, part of the formal local government structure; they are bodies which attempt to articulate the views of local residents and represent them to other parts of the political process. This may be on the basis of common residence (for example, residents' associations) but it may also be on the basis of particular client groups (such as the elderly, or parents of handicapped children) or particular interests held in common (such as being affected by a planning decision). It was this form of organization which Philip Abrams referred to when talking of 'modern neighbourhoodism' being an attempt to *create* a local social world through political action.

The limits of such an approach need to be borne in mind. Uncritical adoption of 'community action' or 'neighbourhood power' is not primarily what is referred to. Rather, it is the articulation of outlooks and interests at a district level, in different forms, which enables the voice of the citizen to be heard at the local level. Formal organizations of all types, including those concerned with care, tend to regard such bodies as a nuisance. Just as local councils look askance at tenants' associations and doctors at Community Health Councils, so local authority Social Service departments will not necessarily welcome district level bodies representing particular client groups or interest groups. Yet unless such developments are fostered it will be difficult to give real meaning to the 'interweaving' of formal and informal care. In the absence of such developments it is likely to continue to remain very much a pious aspiration.

7

The Future of
Informal Care

What of the future of 'community care'? It is time to draw some of the threads of the preceding discussion together, pinpointing failures in policy and drawing some conclusions. It is unlikely that government policy will change very much in the short term. The policy-making process involves too many conflicting pressures; politicians and officials tend to be wedded to small, incremental changes, so that new initiatives reached on the basis of rational knowledge are the exception rather than the rule (cf. Bulmer, 1986b). Nevertheless, significant shifts in policy are occurring. The closure of large hospitals for the mentally handicapped and mentally ill is a good case in point. It began in the United States and has only recently gathered momentum in Britain.

FOUR LACUNAE

For a policy to be enunciated and implemented is one thing; to assess its effects is quite another. In assessing the effects of government policies for 'community care', four major lacunae are evident in Britain.

The first lacuna is the lack of any consistent family policy or attempt to spell out policies for the provision of social support to the family by the state. This is not to say that state action has not impinged in profound ways upon the family, but the family has been assumed to be a part of the private realm, so that policies have not been directly framed to affect the family. Policies, for example, for the taxation of married women or for the income support of low-income families have not been framed explicitly with the family in mind, and indeed in the 1970s this led to the introduction of a specific benefit, Family Income Supplement, designed to fill some of the gaps left by this indirect approach. The assumptions underlying these indirect policies have reflected long-established patterns of dependency within families and a long-established division of labour between the sexes. Thus, for example, female breadwinners have been treated much less favourably within the social security system, and in a variety of ways, than male breadwinners (Land and Parker, 1978).

The lack of any explicit family policy has impinged sharply upon the provision of social care, and is a partial explanation of why 'community care' as it is implemented is in many ways so vague and lacking in focus. The effective government attitude to social care over a long period of time has been either that the ordinary, informal family system will provide care and support, possibly bolstered by neighbours or friends, with some minor professional support, or that the state will assume major or complete responsibility for the care of the dependent, as when, for example, an elderly person enters an old people's home or a patient is admitted to a mental hospital. The latter is only likely to happen when the family's ability to care has diminished through death or incapacity, or where the problems faced are so severe that professional help is required. One consequence has been that British social services have treated classes of persons in need (for example, the elderly) or categories of disease (for example, the mentally ill) rather than families.

The roles of the family in providing care has been seen, as regards official policy, as precarious, easily upset by too much radical state intervention within an essentially private realm. Official policy acts both as a check on families abdicating their responsibilities and prevents an uncontrollable upsurge of demand for support which the state cannot provide. Thus, over a long period, 'state help with the personal [caring] tasks under-taken by family members, notably women [has been] defined as exceptional or else disguised as something which is not easily generalizable to a wide spectrum of family roles and tasks: for example, as education, medical treatment, or 'community care' (Land and Parker, 1978, p. 360). Official policy, despite the rhetoric of 'community care' in recent years, maintains this position, evident in government resistance to campaigns to extend social security payments to various classes of the disabled and housebound or their carers. The vacuum at the heart of 'community care' policy derives from the assumption that, in the majority of cases of quite diverse kinds of need, the family will provide from its own resources. To over-simplify, in some areas of provision 'community care' can, in effect, mean unsupported family care. And the family members who provide that care are, of course, women.

The second lacuna is the failure to develop a policy to support women acting as informal carers. The scope of the tending care and material and psychological support provided by an estimated $1\frac{1}{4}$ million women in contemporary Britain is hardly recognized by government. Few of these women receive any financial support for the work that they do; they are entitled to little or no fiscal relief through tax allowances; and services to those that they care for are often reduced or withdrawn because an informal carer is available to offer help. The burdens borne vary, but for the more exigent types of material support and tending, for example, with the elderly mentally confused or the severely handicapped, these can be very onerous indeed (cf. Lewis, 1986). To a very large extent, this social contribution is not recognized in government policy-making for 'community care'. Moreover, the medium-term plans of government (to the extent that it has any) seem to take no notice of the demographic estimates of numbers of supporters who are relatives available at the end of this century, quoted in Chapter 1, which have major implications for the availability of informal care from kin. 'Community care' cannot be ridden on the backs of women relatives indefinitely, and certain social trends – geographical mobility, increases in married women's activity rates, the growth in divorce and the reconstitution of families – are tending to reduce the availability of care from such informal sources. Greater attention to these trends, and to the implications of women bearing the brunt of informal care, is required on the part of policy-makers (cf. Finch, 1984).

The policy for ex-mental patients clearly exemplifies a third lacuna, the failure to think through the implications for *informal* care of the de-institutionalization of the mentally ill and mentally handicapped. The closure of large institutions has proceeded apace in Britain in recent years, and is still continuing. Policy provision for discharged inmates has focused on, first, the provision of housing and sheltered accommodation, and secondly, the provision of *formal* care *in* the community through day centers, outpatient access, G.P. support, psychiatric nursing services, and so on. There has been very little attention paid to the implications of the policy for informal care and carers, though the policy's impact is considerable. In many respects, the problems arising are greater than those with the dependent elderly, for although the numbers involved are smaller, some of those affected present more disturbed behaviour which is more difficult for an untrained and unqualified informal carer (usually a member of the family) to cope with. Such issues have been brushed under the carpet as the blueprint for the dismantling of the large Victorian mental institutions has been proceeded with, though the Audit Commission (1986) has recently produced a withering analysis of financial failures of co-ordination and planning. There are good reasons for pursuing the current policy, but its implications for care of the ex-patients by the community have not been adequately followed-through.

The fourth lacuna in official policies for community care reflects the third lacuna, but writ large. The lack of serious attention to the feasibility of 'interweaving' formal and informal care is exemplified by the assumption that, for some ex-patients at least, there will be informal carers available and willing to take on some responsibility for the person to be cared for. The discussion in the last chapter demonstrated the manifest problems which there are in trying to mesh formal and informal care. To take but one example: what criteria are to be used in delivering home help services to housebound elderly people who also receive support from informal carers? Too often the rules according to which service is provided render formal and informal care alternatives rather than complementary care. The succession of care described in the case on p. 176 is much more common than genuine complementarity. The government is aware of the problem and the need to plan for such complementarity. Complementarity was the central recommendation of the Barclay Committee's report on the tasks of social workers, and in September 1984 the Secretary of State for Social Services envisaged a new role for local authority social service departments based on 'interweaving'. Yet neither initiative has led to much change, and the latter seems to be suspended because of intractable political and intellectual difficulties (cf. Bulmer, 1986c). It is too easy for policy-makers to make facile assumptions about the availability of normal carers, and to treat informal care as, in effect, a 'black box'. Much closer attention is required both to what is going on within the box, and to how the interface between formal and informal care can be adjusted and fitted together.

INTELLECTUAL AND POLICY CONFUSIONS

These four lacunae in the realm of policy can be linked directly to the intellectual confusions, discussed in earlier chapters, that underly policy confusions. The use of the term 'community' is a prime case in point. 'Community care' policy is a shambles, in part because 'community' has become a vacuous term, meaning all things to all people. It is very difficult to give the term consistent and useful meaning, yet it goes on being used because of its powerful and evocative reference. Even alternative terminology, notably 'social networks', tends to be used in a loose, metaphorical, and sometimes meaningless way, and becomes a truism or a tautology (we all have informal social ties of some sort) rather than a useful tool in analyzing the provision and potential of informal social care.

There is similar confusion about the philosophical and social bases of care discussed in Chapter 5. Official pronouncements tend to assume that obligation, duty and altruism are the principal factors in the provision of informal care, the first two displayed within the family, the latter, altruism, pre-eminently in the voluntary sector. Yet this is a gross over-simplification, ignoring in the first place the role played by tradition, particularly the personal ties between those who have lived together for a long period, and, more generally, neglecting the important part which reciprocity and exchange play in the construction and maintenance of social obligations. Awareness of these factors has yet to permeate official pronouncements on informal care. The extent to which the voluntary sector relies on beneficence, rather than altruism, is also not adequately understood, with the consequent social distance between volunteer and person cared for often interfering in the effectiveness or acceptability of the help offered. Indeed, to the extent that voluntary care is bureaucratized (as in WRVS and Meals on Wheels) it becomes a type of formal care rather than informal care.

The final intellectual confusion underlying policy is the failure to think through clearly what it is, for particular client groups in particular circumstances, that supports care. Is it love? Is it duty? Is it a desire to reciprocate services rendered? Is it the existence of the necessary organizational infrastructure? Is it the existence of financial rewards for carers? Is it the existence of fiscal benefits for carers and/or cared for? The whole policy discussion of community care is confused in this respect, partly because for too long informal care (particularly by kin) has been treated as 'natural', resting on love or duty, and treated as essentially unproblematical. Yet if it has shown one thing, it is to be hoped that this book has made it clear that informal care cannot be taken for granted. Its appearance is not automatic. It has to be worked at. Policy-makers need to devote much more attention to the conditions which can promote informal care, particularly those which are within the control of the policy-maker. More will be said of this below.

These intellectual confusions, then, go some way to explain the uncertainties and vagaries of 'community care' as a social policy. They are unlikely to be resolved by pursuing a nirvana of terminological exactitude, much though that might commend itself to fastidious social scientists. A more fruitful way forward is to try to extract some tentative generalizations from earlier chapters which may serve to clarify the nature of 'community' and local attachments and provide a sounder basis for policy than the present appeal to resonant, but vacuous, terms.

CONCLUDING GENERALIZATIONS

The first clear conclusion is that policies which postulate a single local 'community' or neighbourhood through which care is to be provided are unlikely to be viable. Such bounded localities are largely a thing of the past, and the critical analytic questions concern the extent to which people's social networks are maintained within the locality or outside it. This is an empirical question, the answer to which should not be prejudged. Policies which focus purely upon the local community become, of necessity, partial and restricted in scope. The significant personal ties of local residents – above all though not exclusively with kin – lie as much outside the locality as within it.

A second most significant observation is that to deliver formal caring services – such as 'patch' social work or neighbourhood nursing or home help services – at a local level provides no guarantee that they will mesh more easily, if at all, with informal caring in the locality. There is a good deal of evidence to show that the imperatives of organizations too easily become their overriding concerns, and that co-ordination and liaison with outside individuals and bodies becomes of secondary importance. Local delivery of formal services does not necessarily overcome any more effectively the obstacles to 'interweaving' identified earlier, whatever the rhetorical claims of 'localism' as a policy.

It is unlikely that the terminology of community will wither away in public discourse. Given this, the best social scientists can do is to reiterate the theme that the existence of patterns of local social relations needs to be investigated, not taken as given, *a priori*, and to propose more realistic models of the nature of such local social relations. Of the three models considered in earlier chapters, the Simmel-Wirth image of 'community lost' in single-stranded personal ties has not found much support. Nor does the contrary picture of 'community regained', of *gemeinschaft* within *gesellschaft*, of urban villages within the metropolitan region, accurately portray modern community life. The most satisfactory model, though, in urgent need of further refinement and extension, would seem to be that of 'community liberated'. Modern urban dwellers, supported by the motor car and the telephone, have more widely dispersed personal ties than those within the immediate locality, particularly among kin and friends. This is shown most vividly in Willmott's estimate (1986a, p. 27) that five out of six British families participate in either a dispersed extended family or a dispersed kinship network, in which members are not locally co-resident and, that although the dispersed extended family may meet frequently, this involves travel from some distance. The importance of this attri-tion of locally based attachments for 'community care' policies cannot be exaggerated. For a considerable proportion of the population, the street or neighbourhood is the place in which they live, but their most significant informal social relationships are not, in general, with their co-residents.

A linked concept which helps to reinforce the changing nature of local attachments is the idea of the community of limited liability. People do form local attachments and identify with particular areas, but more usually for specific reasons because they share social characteristics with others (such as being parents of young children at the local primary school) or are the object of official action (for example, local residents in whose area it is proposed to open a mental handicap hostel). These attachments of a limited kind to the local community are not *gemeinschaftlich* but are based upon age, stage in the life cycle and choice on the part of those who participate. The community of limited liability, from the standpoint of community care, may be negative as well as positive. This is particularly apparent in relation to policies to run-down large mental institutions. Local residents, even if they favour the policy in general terms, tend to be markedly unenthusiastic if it is proposed to establish small residential units for ex-patients suffering either from mental illness or mental handicap in their own areas. Such opposition is not universal, and the results depend upon local planning controls, but it appears to rest to a considerable extent upon fear of unpredictability and stereotypes of patient behaviour which have little basis in reality. This underlines the point once again that in many people's minds, and according to official policy, community care means care by the families of those in need of care, not some wider conception of social responsibility. The value of the concept of community of limited liability is a reminder that, outside the personal ties with kin and friends, the responsibilities for others which people acknowledge tend to be narrow and fairly specific, not broad and universal.

The role of voluntary action should not be lost sight of. In the neighbourhood case field, for example, voluntary care of an informal kind has made a far from negligible impact. Voluntary care ranges from extensions of informal care, as in 'good neigh-bour' schemes, to quite highly organized provision of formal care

which in many respects resembles statutory care. Some services –
Meals on Wheels is a notable example – are provided in some areas
by statutory services and in some areas by voluntary services.
Voluntary social services play a distinctive role (cf. Brenton,
1985), but they are not able to provide universal services in the
way that government can. In part, this is a matter of resources,
but even more of manpower and the availability of volunteers. In
Britain there is a marked class bias in the availability of volunteers. They are much more forthcoming in middle-class areas,
which are not, of course, the areas of greatest social need. Moreover there is some evidence, which has been discussed in Chapter
5, that beneficence and altruism are being displaced by reciprocity
as prime motivating factors in voluntary action. Whatever some
politicians wishing to reduce the role of statutory services may
believe, voluntary effort cannot provide the solution to the
demand for social care. 'It is inconceivable that return to volunteer service is the answer for modern industrial society' (Karl,
1984, p. 520).

The idea that voluntary effort promotes public participation in
general also needs to be critically examined, for it has little
substance. Given the strata of society from which volunteers are
drawn, it is likely that they will tend to represent particular points
of view. In the WRVS, for example, members of the Church of
England and supporters of the Conservative party are strongly
represented. Such voluntary effort may thus be an effective way
of expressing at a local level the views and interests of particular
sections of society, but it should not be confused with a move
towards greater public participation (Brenton, 1985). From the
point of view of involving a cross-section of the public in both
care and participation, self-help groups are a much more promis-
ing means of social engineering. Drawing to a much greater
extent upon self-interest and reciprocity, they are nevertheless a
way of providing genuine mutual support and aid to cared-for
and carers (often with severe difficulties), and at the same time
they articulate the interests of that particular group to the wider
community.

What self-help groups do not articulate, however, is a broader
public interest. For that to be achieved, some have argued the case
for greater degrees of neighbourhood political action, most notably in the 'local control' movement in the United States. Local

action to push local interests, including the provision of care, is certainly one way in which participation may be fostered. The current vogue for decentralization in some English local authorities is a related phenomenon, although it is doubtful whether change in the formal organization of local government will necessarily of itself bring formal and informal care any closer together. Fostering local participation is important, but given the model of community liberated in terms of which we are operating, it is unlikely to be the nirvana it is sometimes represented to be.

These tentative sociological conclusions require much further elaboration and empirical testing, but they at least act as a counter to traditional, unreflective notions of 'community' which have little basis in contemporary reality. In what directions do the conclusions point the policy-maker seeking to provide care in and by the community? The following suggestions are necessarily somewhat prescriptive, and readers may arrive at other conclusions to those which follow. They are, however, based on the preceding analysis, and seek to take account of contemporary social care as it exists today.

The main conclusion is an obvious one, but worth reiterating. Formal and informal care are not substitutes for each other, but complementary. It is inadequate to rely upon one or the other alone; both are needed for effective provision for need. Several considerations point to this conclusion. On the one hand, there are clearly finite limits to the amount of care which statutory services can provide, reflected in the rather stringent rules which apply both to social security benefits for various classes of dependent person and in service delivery (for example, entitlement to home-help service). If officially provided care is not paid for, then rationing devices of a more or less explicit kind must be used. On the other hand, the capacity of informal carers to cope may be becoming more limited in some respects. Demographic change, economic change and greater geographic mobility, may mean fewer carers available within the family. With medical advances, some types of dependency (for example, among the very elderly infirm, or among some types of mental handicap) may become more common while, at the same time, these types of dependency become more difficult for a lay carer to deal with (for instance, the great stress which may be associated with looking after a demented elderly person). Recognizing these pressures in both directions, what is urgently required are more creative explorations along the boundary between formal and informal care. Despite the rhetoric of 'interweaving', sharing care and complementarity, there are relatively few examples of successful combinations of the two which endure for any length of time.

Truism though it is, one of the first targets must be intra- and inter-organizational boundaries in the personal caring fields. Within social services departments, home-help services and social work teams are too insulated from each other. Within local health services, district nurses, health visitors and general practitioner services are run too much in parallel, without adequate co-ordination. Social services as a whole, and health services as a whole, are largely ineffective in co-ordinating their activities, a proposition which is being demonstrated once again in the closure of large mental institutions. The conclusion of the Audit Commission (1986) on these issues, and their recommendations for a common basic training for community care workers deserve serious study.

More exploration is needed about providing informal care through the formal system. Policy-makers need not be squeamish about using money to promote care. There are various models. Local care managers may be given budgets out of which they may purchase a package of personal care for their clients (cf. Challis and Davies, 1980). Local authorities may employ locally recruited staff to provide care and support, such as home helps and street wardens, who provide some of the support in a world of community liberated which in the past came from kin or neighbours. In the case of the elderly, mentally ill and mentally handicapped, there is considerable scope for employing trained auxiliary staff who are neither highly skilled nor particularly highly paid but who provide tending and material support to those in need. Paradoxically, payment appears to appeal to feelings of reciprocity. Those in receipt of care are less worried about being given something for nothing if they know that the person helping them is being paid for doing so. On the other hand, levels of payment for this type of care is a difficult issue, and schemes making only nominal payment invite criticism for providing care on the cheap.

Greater sensitivity is needed among policy-makers to the delicate world of informal care, to the fragile balance inherent in some caring relationships (for example, between neighbours), the emotional loading (both positive and negative) in kinship ties, and to the lines which people themselves draw around their private worlds. More thought is needed about the means of access to those in need of support, and, in particular, to ways of considering with family members means of supporting both cared-for and carers. In a world where kin are the predominant source of care, the uncritical enthusiasm for community social work and 'natural helping networks' seems somewhat misplaced, given all the pitfalls which lie in its path. At the least there is doubt whether fully effective informal care can be provided only by non-kin, without formal sector involvement.

The creative exploration of the role of the family in care would involve an explicit attempt on the part of policy-makers to provide some supporting services so that collaboration in care rather than succession became more common. This would involve recognition of the changing role, and economic situation, of women. It would require changes in the treatment of married women, the physically disabled and the very dependent in the tax, national insurance and social security systems. (To give one example, in parts of Eastern Europe women who remain at home to look after an elderly relative are credited with notional contributions to the state insurance scheme, even though they are not at work.) It would involve much more careful assessment of the burdens of caring on carers, and attempts to relieve some of those physical and emotional burdens through government-provided services (such as respite care). This is already done to some extent through day centres. At present these issues are not addressed directly. Current government policy tends to be minimalist – put as much of the onus upon the family as possible in the circumstances, minimising government involvement – without ever addressing directly the issue of how collaboration between formal and informal services may be fostered.

One final suggestion may also be worth pursuing. Already in the mental health field the idea of a 'key-worker', who has particular responsibility for the management of the care of an ex-patient discharged into the community, is quite widely used. The key worker might be a psychiatrist or G.P., or more probably a community psychiatric nurse or social worker. Given the likely continuing fragmentation or different services, with all the problems to which this gives rise, the idea of a 'key-worker' to co-ordinate care has considerably wider applicability to the care of the infirm elderly and disabled. Barclay's conception of the social work role is similar, although there is no reason why the key-worker need be a social worker: he or she could, for example, be a home help organizer, or a district nurse. There is great scope here for greater collaboration within and between formal services, and between formal provision and informal carers, though those involved would need to be trained for the task and some of the obstacles identified in Chapter 6 tackled at source.

Community care policy is a vital challenge as the twentieth century draws to a close. Effective community care is part and parcel of meeting the needs of dependent members of society. Yet, as earlier chapters have shown, it is a policy area particularly prone to vagueness, confusion and misconceptions. At the heart there is a vacuum. While day-to-day care by both formal carers and informal supporters goes on, much more serious thought needs to be given to framing policies which will shape the pattern of provision in the early twenty-first century. The suggestions offered at the end of this chapter are put forward with that end in view, and to stimulate debate.

References

Abrams, M. (1978), *Beyond Three Score Years and Ten* (London: Age Concern).

Abrams, P. (1978a), 'Community care, some research problems and priorities', in Barnes and Connelly (eds.) (1978), pp. 78–99.

Abrams, P. (1978b), *Neighbourhood Care and Social Policy: A Research Perspective* (Berkhamsted, Hertfordshire: The Volunteer Centre).

Abrams, P. (1978c), 'Towns and economic growth: some theories and problems', in P. Abrams and E. A. Wrigley (eds.), *Towns in Societies: Essays in Economic History and Historical Sociology* (Cambridge: Cambridge University Press), pp. 9–33.

Abrams, P. (1980), 'Social change, social networks and neighbourhood care', *Social Work Service*, 22 February, pp. 12–23.

Abrams, P. (1984), 'Realities of Neighbourhood Care: the interactions between statutory, voluntary and informal social care', *Policy and Politics*, vol. 12, no. 4, pp. 413–29.

Abrams, P., Abrams, S., Humphrey, R. and Snaith, R. (1981), *Action for Care: A Review of Good Neighbour Schemes in England* (Berkhamsted, Hertfordshire: The Volunteer Centre).

Abrams, P., Abrams, S., Humphrey, R. and Snaith, R. (1986), *Patterns of Neighbourhood Care* (Durham: University of Durham, Department of Sociology and Social Policy, Rowntree Research Unit).

Allan, G. (1979), *A Sociology of Friendship and Kinship* (London: Allen & Unwin).

Allan, G. A. (1983), 'Informal networks of care: issues raised by Barclay', *British Journal of Social Work*, vol. 13, pp. 417–33.

Allan, G. (1985), *Family Life* (Oxford: Basil Blackwell).

Anderson, M. (1971), *Family Structure in Nineteenth Century Lancashire* (Cambridge: Cambridge University Press).

Archbishop of Canterbury's Commission (1985), *Faith In The City: A Call for Action by Church and Nation* (London: Church House Publishing).

Aries, P. (1962), *Centuries of Childhood* (New York: Knopf).

Arrow, K. J. (1972), 'Gifts and exchanges', *Philosophy and Public Affairs*, vol. 1, no. 4, summer, pp. 343–62.

Audit Commission (1986), *Making a Reality of Community Care* (London: HMSO).

Babchuk, N. (1965), 'Primary friends and kin: a study of the associations of middle class couples', *Social Forces*, vol. 43, pp. 483–93.

Babchuk, N. and Bates, A. (1963), 'The primary relations of middle class couples', *American Sociological Review*, vol. 28, pp. 377–91.

Bailey, F. G. (ed.) (1971), *Gifts and Poisons: the politics of reputation* (Oxford: Blackwell).

Ball, C. and Ball, M. (1982), *What the Neighbours Say: a report on a study of neighbours* (Berkhamsted, Hertfordshire: The Volunteer Centre).

Barclay Report, the (1982), *Social Workers: Their Role and Tasks* (Report of a working party under the chairmanship of Mr P. M. Barclay) (London: Bedford Square Press).

Barker, J. (1980), 'The Relationship of "Informal" Care to "Formal" Social Services: who helps people deal with social and health problems if they arise in old age?', in S. Lonsdale *et al.* (eds.), *Teamwork in the British and American Social Services: British and American Perspectives* (London: Croom Helm), pp. 159–80.

Barnes, J. A. (1954), 'Class and committees in a Norwegian island parish', *Human Relations*, vol. 7, pp. 39–58.

Barnes, J. A. and Harary, F. (1983), 'Graph theory in network analysis', *Social Networks*, vol. 5, pp. 235–44.

Barnes, J. H. and Connelly, N. (eds.) (1978), *Social Care Research* (London: Policy Studies Institute and Bedford Square Press).

British Association of Social Workers (1971), *Confidentiality in Social Work* (London: British Association of Social Workers).

Bates, A. (1964), 'Privacy: a useful concept?', *Social Forces*, vol. 42, pp. 429–34.

Bates, A. P. and Babchuk, N. (1961), 'The Primary Group: a reappraisal', *The Sociological Quarterly*, vol. 1, pp. 181–91.

Bayley, M. J. (1973), *Mental Handicap and Community Care* (London: Routledge & Kegan Paul).

Bayley, M. J. (1982), 'Helping Care to Happen in the Community', in A. Walker (ed.), *Community Care: The Family, the State and Social Policy* (Oxford: Blackwell), pp. 179–96.

Bayley, M. J., Seyd, R., Tennant, A. and Parker, P. (1984), *Neighbourhood Services Project: Dinnington: Working Papers* (Sheffield: University of Sheffield Department of Sociological Studies).

Becker, G. (1981), *A Treatise on the Family: the Economic Approach* (Cambridge, Mass.: Harvard University Press).

Becker, L. C. (1986), *Reciprocity* (London: Routledge & Kegan Paul).

Bell, C. (1968), *Middle Class Families* (London: Routledge & Kegan Paul).

Bell, C. and McKee, L. (1984), 'His unemployment, her problem' (Birmingham: University of Aston, mimeo).

Bell, C. and Newby, H. (1971), *Community Studies* (London: Allen & Unwin).

Bell, D. (1956), 'The Theory of Mass Society', *Commentary*, July.

Bender, T. (1978), *Community and Social Change in America* (New Brunswick, N.J: Rutgers University Press).

Benney, M., Weiss, R., Meyersohn, R. and Riesman, D. (1959). 'Christmas is an apartment hotel', *American Journal of Sociology*, vol. 65, no. 3, pp. 233–40.

Beresford, P. and Croft, S. (1986), *Whose Welfare? a study and practical guide to changing social services* (Brighton: Lewis Cohen Urban Studies Centre).

Berger, B. (1960), *Working Class Suburb: a study of auto workers in suburbia* (Berkeley: University of California Press).

Berger, P. L. (1980), 'In praise of particularity: the concept of mediating structures', in P. L. Berger, *Facing Up to Modernity: excursions in society, politics and religion* (New York: Basic Books), pp. 130–41.

Berger, P. L. and Neuhaus, R. J. (1977), *To Empower People: the role of mediating structures in public policy* (Washington, DC: American Enterprise Institute).

Berkman, L. and Syme, L. (1979), 'Social networks, host resistance and mortality', *American Journal of Epidemiology*, vol. 109, pp. 187–204.

Blackstone, W. (1783), *Commentaries on the laws of England* (London: Strahan).

Blau, P. M. (1963), *The Dynamics of Bureaucracy* (Chicago: University of Chicago Press).

Blau, P. M. (1964), *Exchange and Power in Social Life* (New York: Wiley).

Blau, Z. S. (1973), *Old Age in a Changing Society* (New York: Franklin Watts).

Bloch, M. (1962), *Feudal Society* (London: Routledge & Kegan Paul).

Boissevain, J. (1974), *Friends of Friends: Networks, Manipulators and Coalitions* (Oxford: Blackwell).

Boissevain, J. (1979), 'Network analysis: a reappraisal', *Current Anthropology*, vol. 20, pp. 392–4.

Boissevain, J. (1985), 'Networks', in A. and J. Kuper (eds.), *The Social Science Encyclopedia* (London: Routledge & Kegan Paul), pp. 557–8.

Bok, S. (1984), *Secrets: on the ethics of concealment and revelation* (Oxford: Oxford University Press).

Booth, A. and Hess, E. (1974), 'Cross-sexual friendships', *Journal of Marriage and the Family*, vol. 36, pp. 38–47.

Bott, E. (1957), *Family and Social Network* (London: Tavistock) (Revised edition with new introduction, 1971).

Bracey, H. E. (1964), *Neighbours* (London: Routledge & Kegan Paul).

Brenton, M. (1985), *The Voluntary Sector in the British Social Services* (London: Longman).

Briggs, A. and Oliver, J. (eds.) (1985), *Caring: experiences of looking after disabled relatives* (London: Routledge & Kegan Paul).

Brown, G. W. and Harris, T. (1978), *The Social Origins of Depression: A Study of Psychiatric Disorder in Women* (London: Tavistock).

Bulmer, J. (1986), Personal communication.

Bulmer, M. (1986a), *Neighbours: the work of Philip Abrams* (Cambridge: Cambridge University Press).

Bulmer, M. (1986b), *Social Science and Social Policy* (London: Allen & Unwin).

Bulmer, M. (1986c), 'Can caring come together?', *New Society* 4 July, pp. 18–20.

Bulmer, M. (1987), 'Privacy and confidentiality as obstacles to inter-weaving formal and informal care', *Journal of Voluntary Action Research*, forthcoming.

Bulmer, M. (ed.) (1975), *Working Class Images of Society* (London: Routledge & Kegan Paul).

Bulmer, M. (ed.) (1977), *Mining and Social Change: Durham County in the Twentieth Century* (London: Croom Helm).

Bulmer, M. (ed.) (1978), *Social Policy Research* (London: Macmillan).

Cantor, M. H. (1979), 'Neighbours and friends: an overlooked resource in the informal support system', *Research on Aging*, vol. 1, no. 4, pp. 434–63.

Caplan, G. (1974), 'Support systems', in G. Caplan (ed.), *Support Systems and Community Mental Health: lectures on concept development* (New York: Behavioral Publications), pp. 1–40.

Cassell, J. (1974), 'Psychosocial processes and "stress": theoretical formulations', *International Journal of Health Services*, vol. 4, pp. 471–82.

Castells, M. (1968), 'Y-a-t-il une sociologie urbaine?', *Sociologie du Travail*, vol. 1, pp. 72–90, Translated as 'Is there an urban sociology?' in C. G. Pickvance (ed.), *Urban Sociology: Critical Essays* (London: Tavistock, 1976), pp. 33–50.

Castells, M. (1977), *The Urban Question* (London: Edward Arnold).

Challis, D. and Davies, B. (1980), 'A new approach to community care for the elderly', *British Journal of Social Work*, vol. 10, pp. 1–18.

Chappel, N. L. (1983), 'Informal support networks among the elderly', *Research on Aging*, vol. 5, no. 1, March, pp. 77–99.

Chinoy, E. (1955), *Automobile Workers and the American Dream* (Garden City, NY: Doubleday).

Chrisman, N. J. and Kleinman, A. (1983), 'Popular health care, social networks and cultural meanings', in D. Mechanic (ed.), *Handbook of Health, Health Care and the Health Professions* (New York: Free Press).

Clarke, M. (1982), 'Where is the Community Which Cares?', *British Journal of Social Work*, vol. 12, pp. 453–69.

Collard, D. (1978), *Altruism and Economy: a study of non-selfish economics* (Oxford: Martin Robertson).

Collins, A. H. and Pancoast, D. L. (1976), *Natural Helping Networks: A Strategy for Prevention* (Washington, DC: National Association of Social Workers).

Collison, P. (1963), *The Cutteslowe Walls* (London: Faber & Faber).

Cooley, C. H. (1909), *Social Organisation: a study of the larger mind* (New York: Scribner's).

Coward, R. T. (1982), 'Cautions about the role of natural helping networks in programs for the rural elderly', in N. Stinnet *et al.* (eds.), *Family Strengths 4: Positive Support Systems* (Lincoln, Nebraska: University of Nebraska Press), pp. 291–307.

D'Abbs, P. (1982), *Social Support Networks: a Critical Review of Models and Findings* (Melbourne: Institute of Family Studies Monograph no. 1).

Darvill, G. (1983), 'Shuttle Diplomacy in the Personal Social Services:

interweaving statutory and informal care in a changing Britain', in D. L. Pancoast *et al.* (eds.), (1983), pp. 239–60.

Daunton, M. J. (1983), 'Public place and private space: the Victorian city and the working-class household', in D. Fraser and A. Sutcliffe (eds.), *The Pursuit of Urban History* (London: Edward Arnold), pp. 212–33.

Deakin, N. (1986), 'Formal structures and their relation to community', in P. Willmott (ed.) (1986), pp. 31–40.

Dennis, N. (1958), 'The popularity of the neighbourhood community idea', *Sociological Review*, vol. 6, no. 2, December, pp. 191–206.

Dennis, N. (1963), 'Who needs neighbours?', *New Society*, vol. 2, no. 43, 25 July, pp. 8–11.

Dennis, N., Henriques, F. and Slaughter, C. (1956), *Coal is Our Life* (London: Eyre & Spottiswoode).

Derlega, V. J. and Margulis, S. Y. (1982), 'Why loneliness occurs: the interrelationship of social-psychological and privacy concepts', in Peplau and Perlman (1982), pp. 152–65.

Dexter, M. and Harbert, W. (1983), *The Home Help Service* (London: Tavistock).

Department of Health and Social Security (1978), 'The D.H.S.S. Perspective' in Barnes and Connelly (1978), pp. 1–44.

Department of Health and Social Security (1981a), *Care in the Community: A Consultative Document on Moving Resources for Care in England* (London: DHSS).

Department of Health and Social Security (1981b), *Care in Action* (London: HMSO).

Department of Health and Social Security (1981c), *Growing Older*, Cmnd. 8173 (London: HMSO).

Department of Health and Social Security (1986), *Neighbourhood Nursing: A Focus for Care* (The Cumberlege Report) (London: HMSO).

Dickinson, F. G. (ed.) (1962), *Philanthropy and Public Policy* (New York: National Bureau of Economic Research).

Donnison, D. (1967), *The Government of Housing* (Harmondsworth: Penguin).

Dore, R. P. (1958), *City Life in Japan: A Study of a Tokyo Ward* (London: Routledge & Kegan Paul).

Dore, R. P. (1983), 'Goodwill and the spirit of market capitalism', *British Journal of Sociology*, vol. 34, pp. 459–82.

Drake, A. W., Finkelstein, F. N. and Sapolsky, H. M. (1982), *The American Blood Supply* (Cambridge, Mass.: MIT).

Drake, St. Clair and Cayton, H. (1945), *Black Metropolis: A Study of Negro Life in a Northern City* (New York: Harcourt Brace).

Duesenberry, J. S. (1960), 'Comment' in Universities – National Bureau Committee for Economic Research, *Demographic and Economic Change in Developed Countries* (Princeton, NJ: Princeton University Press), pp. 231–4.

Durkheim, E. (1933), *The Division of Labor in Society* (New York: Free Press) (first published in French 1893).

Durkheim, E. (1952), *Suicide: a study in sociology* (London: Routledge & Kegan Paul) (first published in French 1897).

Elder, G. H. and Rockwell, R. C. (1979), 'The life course and human development', *International Journal of Behavioural Development*, vol. 2, pp. 1–21.

Ell, K. (1984), 'Social networks, social support and health: a review', *Social Service Review*, vol. 58, March, pp. 133–49.

Elshtain, J. B. (1981), *Public Man, Private Woman* (Oxford: Martin Robertson).

Equal Opportunity Commission (1982), *Who Cares for the Carers? Opportunities for those caring for the elderly and handicapped* (Manchester: EOC).

Ericksen, E. and Yancey, W. L. (1977), 'The locus of strong ties' (unpublished MS, Department of Sociology, Temple University).

Eversley, D. (1982), 'Some new aspects of ageing in Britain', in T. K. Hareven and K. J. Adams (eds.), *Ageing and Life Course Transitions: an Interdisciplinary Perspective* (New York: Guildford Press), pp. 245–65.

Family Policy Studies Centre (1984), *The Forgotten Army: family care and elderly people* (London: Family Policy Studies Centre).

Festinger, L., Schachter, S. and Back, K. (1950), *Social Pressures in Informal Groups* (New York: Harper).

Finch, J. (1984), 'Community care: developing non-sexist alternatives', *Critical Social Policy*, Vol. 9, spring, pp. 6–18.

Finch, J. and Groves, D. (1980), 'Community care and the family: a case for equal opportunities?', *Journal of Social Policy*, vol. 9, no. 4, pp. 487–514.

Finch, J. and Groves, D. (eds.) (1983), *A Labour of Love: Women, Work and Caring* (London: Routledge & Kegan Paul).

Firth, R., Hubert, J. and Forge, A. (1970), *Families and their Relatives* (London: Routledge & Kegan Paul).

Fischer, C. S. (1976), *The Urban Experience* (New York: Harcourt Brace Jovanovich).

Fischer, C. S., Jackson, R. M., Stueve, C. A., Gerson, K. and Jones, L. M., with Baldassare, M. (1977), *Networks and Places: social relations in the urban setting* (New York: Free Press).

Fischer, C. S. (1982), *To Dwell Among Friends: Personal Networks in Town and City* (Chicago: University of Chicago Press).

Fischer, C. S. and Phillips, S. L. (1982), 'Who is alone? social characteristics of people with small networks', in Peplau and Perlman (1982), pp. 21–39.

Fortes, M. (1949), *The Web of Kinship among the Tallensi* (Oxford: Oxford University Press).

Frankfurter, D. L., Smith, M. J. and Caro, F. G. (1981), *Family Care of the Elderly* (Lexington, Mass.: D. C. Heath).

Franck, K. A. (1980), 'Friends and strangers: the social experience of urban and non-urban settings', *Journal of Social Issues*, vol. 36, no. 3, pp. 52–71.

Frazier, E. F. (1939), *The Negro Family in the United States* (Chicago: University of Chicago Press).

Friedrichs, R. W. (1960), 'Alter versus ego: an exploratory assessment of altruism', *American Sociological Review*, vol. 25, no. 4, pp. 496–508.

Fried, M. (1973), *The World of the Urban Working Class* (Cambridge, Mass.: Harvard University Press).

Froland, C. (1980), 'Formal and Informal Care: Discontinuities on a Continuum', *Social Service Review*, vol. 54, no. 4, pp. 572–87.

Froland, C., Pancoast, D. L., Chapman, N. J. and Kimboko, P. J. (1981), *Helping Networks and Human Services* (Beverly Hills: Sage).

Froland, C., Parker, P. and Bayley, M. (1980), 'Relating Formal and Informal Sources of Care: reflections on initiatives in England and America' (Sheffield: University of Sheffield Department of Sociological Studies, mimeo).

Gamarnikov, E., Morgan, D., Purvis, J. and Taylorson, D. (eds.) (1983), *The Public and the Private* (London: Heinemann).

Gans, H. (1962), *The Urban Villagers* (New York: Free Press).

Gans, H. (1964), 'Urbanism and suburbanism as ways of life' in A. M. Rose (ed.), *Human Behaviour and Social Processes* (London: Routledge & Kegan Paul), pp. 625–48.

Gans, H. (1967), *The Levittowners* (New York: Pantheon).

Gilligan, C. (1982), *In A Different Voice: Psychological Theory and Women's Development* (Cambridge, Mass.: Harvard University Press).

Gilroy, D. (1982), 'Informal Care: reality behind the rhetoric', *Social Work Service* 30, pp. 9–19.

Glass, R. (1948), *The Social Background of a Plan* (London: Routledge & Kegan Paul).

Glass, R. (1955), 'Urban Sociology in Great Britain', *Current Sociology*, vol. 4, pp. 5–19.

Glendinning, C. (1986), *A Single Door: Social Work with the Families of Disabled Children* (London: Allen & Unwin).

Gluckman, M. (1963), 'Gossip and scandal', *Current Anthropology*, vol. 4, pp. 307–16.

Goldberg, E. M. and Connelly, N. (1982), *The Effectiveness of Social Care for the Elderly* (London: Heinemann Educational Books).

Goldthorpe, J., Lockwood, D., Bechhofer, F. and Platt, J. (1969), *The Affluent Worker in the Class Structure* (Cambridge: Cambridge University Press).

Goodin, R. E. (1985), *Protecting the Vulnerable: A Reanalysis of our Social Responsibilities* (Chicago: University of Chicago Press).

Gore, S. (1978), 'The effect of social support in moderating the health consequences of unemployment', *Journal of Health and Social Behavior*, vol. 19, pp. 157–65.

Gottleib, B. H. (ed.) (1981), *Social Networks and Social Support* (Beverly Hills: Sage).

Gouldner, A. W. (1954), *Patterns of Industrial Bureaucracy* (New York: Free Press).

Gouldner, A. W. (1960), 'The norm of reciprocity: a preliminary statement', *American Sociological Review*, vol. 25, no. 2, pp. 161–78.

Gouldner, A. W. (1973), 'The importance of something for nothing', in A. W. Gouldner, *For Sociology* (London: Allen Lane), pp. 260–99.

Graham, H. (1983), 'Caring: a labour of love', in Finch and Groves (eds.) (1983), pp. 13–30.

Granovetter, M. (1973), 'The strength of weak ties', *American Journal of Sociology*, vol. 78, no. 6, pp. 1360–80.

Granovetter, M. (1974), *Getting a Job: A Study of Contacts and Careers* (Cambridge, Mass.: Harvard University Press).

Granovetter, M. (1983), 'The strength of weak ties: a network theory revisited', in R. Collins (ed.), *Sociological Theory 1983* (San Francisco: Jossey Bass), pp. 201–33.

Graycar, A. (1983), 'Informal, Voluntary and Statutory Services: The Complex Relationship', *British Journal of Social Work*, vol. 13, pp. 379–93.

Green, S., Creese, A. and Kaufert, J. (1979), 'Social Support and Government Policy on Social Services for the Elderly', *Social Policy and Administration*, vol. 13, no. 3, pp. 210–18.

Hadley, R. and McGrath, M. (1984), *When Social Services are Local: The Normanton Experience* (London: Allen & Unwin).

Hadley, R., Webb, A. and Farrell, C. (1976), *Across the Generations* (London: Allen & Unwin).

Hall, A. and Wellman, B. (1985), 'Social networks and social support', in S. Cohen and L. S. Syme (eds.), *Social Support and Health* (Orlando, Florida: Academic Press), pp. 23–41.

Halsey, A. H. (1974), 'Government against poverty in school and community', in D. Wedderburn (ed.), *Poverty, Inequality and Class Structure* (Cambridge: Cambridge University Press), pp. 123–39.

Hammer, M. (1981), 'Social support, social networks and schizophrenia'. *Schizophrenia Bulletin*, vol. 7, pp. 45–56.

Hannerz, U. (1980), *Exploring the City: inquiries toward an urban anthropology* (New York: Columbia University Press).

Harbert, W. (1983), 'The Nature of Community Care', in Harbert and Rogers (1984), pp. 1–11.

Harbert, W. and Rogers, P. (eds.) (1983), *Community-Based Social Care: The Avon Experience* (NCVO Occasional Paper no. 4) (London: Bedford Square Press).

Hareven, T. K. (1982), *Family Time and Industrial Time: the relationship between the family and work in a New England industrial community* (Cambridge: Cambridge University Press).

Harvey, D. (1973), *Social Justice and the City* (London: Edward Arnold).

Hatch, S. (ed.), *Volunteers: Patterns, Meanings and Motives* (Berkhamsted, Hertfordshire: The Volunteer Centre).

Heath, A. (1976), *Rational Choice and Social Exchange: a critique of exchange theory* (Cambridge: Cambridge University Press).

Heppenstall, M. A. (1971), 'Reputation, criticism and information in an Austrian village', in Bailey (ed.) (1971), pp. 139–66.

Hill, D. M. (1978), 'Privacy and social welfare', in J. B. Young (ed.), *Privacy* (Chichester: Wiley), pp. 155–76.

Hillery, G. A. (1955), 'Definitions of community: areas of agreement', *Rural Sociology*, vol. 20, no. 2, pp. 111–23.

Hillery, G. A. (1968), *Communal Organisations: a study of local societies* (Chicago: University of Chicago Press).

Hirsch, B. J. (1981), 'Social networks and the coping process: creating personal communities', in Gottleib (ed.) (1981), pp. 149–70.

Hirsch, F. (1977), *Social Limits to Growth* (London: Routledge & Kegan Paul).

Hoffman, M. L. (1981), 'Is altruism part of human nature?', *Journal of Personality and Social Psychology*, vol. 40, no. 1, pp. 121–37.

Hole, V. (1959), 'Social effects of planned rehousing', *Town Planning Review*, vol. 30, pp. 166–73.

Holmes, A. and Maizels, J. (1979), *Social Workers and Volunteers* (London: British Association of Social Workers).

Homans, G. C. (1961), *Social Behaviour: its elementary forms* (London: Routledge & Kegan Paul).

Hoyt, D. R. and Babchuk, N. (1983), 'Adult kinship networks: the selective formation of intimate ties with kin', *Social Forces*, vol. 62, no. 1, pp. 84–101.

Hunt, A. (1978), *The Elderly At Home: a survey carried out on behalf of the Department of Health and Social Security* (London: HMSO).

Hunter, A. H. (1974), *Symbolic Communities: The Persistence and Change of Chicago's Local Communities* (Chicago: University of Chicago Press).

Hunter, A. H. (1985), 'Private, parochial and public social orders: the problem of crime and incivility in urban communities', in Suttles and Zald (ed.) (1985), pp. 230–42.

Hunter, A. H. and Riger, S. (1986), 'The meaning of community in community mental health', *Journal of Community Psychology*, vol. 14, pp. 55–71.

Hunter, A. H. and Suttles, G. D. (1972), 'The Expanding Community of Limited Liability', in G. D. Suttles, *The Social Construction of Communities* (1972) (Chicago: University of Chicago Press), pp. 44–81.

Jackson, B. and Jackson, S. (1979), *Childminder: a study in action research* (London: Routledge & Kegan Paul).

Jackson, R. M. (1977), 'Social structure and process in friendship choice', in C. S. Fischer et al., *Networks and Places: social relations in the urban setting* (New York: Free Press), pp. 59–78.

Janowitz, M. (1952), *The Community Press in an Urban Setting* (Glencoe, Ill.: Free Press).

Janowitz, M. and Suttles, G. D. (1978), 'The Social Ecology of Citizenship' in R. C. Sarri and Y. Hasenfeld (eds.), *The Management of Human Services* (New York: Columbia University Press), pp. 80–104.

Jerrome, D. (1981), 'The significance of friendship for women in later life', *Ageing and Society*, vol. 1, no. 2, pp. 175–97.

Jerrome, D. (1983), 'Lonely women in a friendship club', *British Journal of Guidance and Counselling*, vol. 11, pp. 10–20.

Jerrome, D. (1984), 'Good company: the sociological implications of friendship', *The Sociological Review*, vol. 32, no. 4, pp. 696–718.

Johnson, M. L. and Cooper, S. (1984), *Informal Care and the Personal Social Services: an interpretive literature review* (London: Policy Studies Institute, mimeo).

Jones, K., Brown, J. and Bradshaw, J. (1978), *Issues in Social Policy* (London: Routledge & Kegan Paul).

Kapferer, B. (1969), 'Norms and the manipulation of relationships in a work context', in J. C. Mitchell (ed.), *Social Networks in Urban Situations: Analyses of Personal Relationships in Central African Towns* (Manchester: Manchester University Press), pp. 181–244.

Kapferer, B. (1972), *Strategy and Transaction in an African Factory: African Workers and Indian Management in a Zambian Town* (Manchester: Manchester University Press).

Karl, B. D. (1984), 'Lo, the poor volunteer: an essay on the relation between history and myth', *Social Service Review*, vol. 58, December, pp. 493–522.

Keller, S. (1968), *The Urban Neighbourhood: a sociological perspective* (New York: Random House).

Keynes, J. M. (1936), *General Theory of Employment, Interest and Money* (London: Macmillan).

Kingston Polytechnic (1972), *The Buxton Report* (Kingston-upon-Thames: Kingston Polytechnic School of Architecture).

Klein, J. (ed.) (1965), *Samples from English Cultures* (London: Routledge & Kegan Paul).

Knight, B. and Hayes, R. (1981), *Self-Help in the Inner City* (London: London Voluntary Services Council).

Knorr-Cetina, K. and Cicourel, A. V. (eds.) (1981), *Advances in Social Theory and Methodology: Towards an Integration of Micro- and Macrosociologies* (London: Routledge & Kegan Paul).

Korman, N. and Glennerster, H. (1985), *Closing a Hospital* (LSE Occasional Papers in Social Administration no. 78) (London: Bedford Square Press).

Krebs, D. L. (1970), 'Altruism: an examination of the concept and a review of the literature', *Psychological Bulletin*, vol. 73, no. 4, pp. 258–302.

Kropotkin, P. (1904), *Mutual Aid: a factor of evolution* (London: Heinemann).

Kuper, L. (1953), 'Blueprint for living together', in L. Kuper (ed.), *Living in Towns* (London: Cressett), pp. 1–202.

Lake, T. (1980), *Loneliness: why it happens and how to overcome it* (London: Sheldon Press).

Land, H. (1978), 'Who Cares for the Family?', *Journal of Social Policy*, vol. 7, no. 3, pp. 357–84.

Land, H. and Parker, R. (1978), 'Family Policy in the United Kingdom', in S. Kamerman and A. Kahn (eds.), *Family Policy: Government and Families in Fourteen Countries* (New York: Columbia University Press), pp. 331–66.

Land, H. and Rose, H. (1985), 'Compulsory altruism for some or an altruistic society for all?', in P. Bean, J. Ferris and D. Whynes (eds.), *In Defence of Welfare* (London: Tavistock), pp. 74–96.

Laumann, E. O. (1973), *Bonds of Pluralism: The Form and Substance of Urban Social Networks* (New York: Wiley).

Laumann, E. O. and Pappi, F. U. (1976), *Networks of Collective Action: A Perspective on Community Influence Systems* (New York: Academic Press).

Leat, D. (1983a), *Getting to Know the Neighbours: a pilot study of the elderly and neighbourly helping* (London: Policy Studies Institute Research Paper 83–2).

Leat, D. (1983b), 'Explaining volunteering: a sociological perspective', in Hatch (ed.) (1983), pp. 51–61.

Leighton, A. H. (1982), *Caring for Mentally Ill People: psychological and social barriers in historical context* (Cambridge: Cambridge University Press).

Lenrow, P. (1978), 'Dilemmas of professional helping: continuities and discontinuities with folk helping roles', in L. Wispé (ed.) (1978), *Altruism, Sympathy and Helping: psychological and sociological principles* (New York: Academic Press), pp. 263–90.

Levin, E., Sinclair, I. and Gorbach, P. (1986), *Families, Services and Confusion in Old Age* (London: Allen & Unwin).

Levine, D. N., Carter, E. B. and Gorman, E. M. (1976), 'Simmel's Influence on American Sociology', *American Journal of Sociology*, vol. 81, pp. 813–45 and 1112–32.

Lewis, J. (1986), *The Caring Process: Mothers and Daughters at Home* (London: LSE Department of Social Science and Administration).

Litwak, E. (1985), *Helping the Elderly: the complementary roles of informal networks and formal systems* (New York: Guilford Press).

Litwak, E. and Meyer, H. J. (1966), 'A Balance Theory of Coordination Between Bureaucratic Organizations and Community Primary Groups', *Administrative Science Quarterly*, vol. 11, no. 1, pp. 31–58.

Litwak, E., Meyer, H. J. and Hollister, C. D. (1977), 'The role of linkage mechanisms between bureaucracies and families', in R. J. Liebert and A. W. Imershein (eds.), *Power, Paradigms and Community Research* (Beverly Hills, Ca.: Sage), pp. 121–52.

Litwak, E. and Szelenyi, I. (1969), 'Primary group structures and their functions: kin, neighbours and friends', *American Sociological Review*, vol. 34, August, pp. 465–81.

Lockwood, D. (1966), 'Sources of variation in working-class images of society', *The Sociological Review*, vol. 14, pp. 249–67.

Lomnitz, L. (1977), *Networks and Marginality: Life in a Mexican Shantytown* (New York: Academic Press).

Lopata, H. Z. (1969), 'Loneliness: forms and components', *Social Problems*, vol. 17, no. 2, pp. 248–62.

Lowenthal, M. F. and Haven, C. (1968), 'Interaction and adaptation: intimacy as a critical variable', *American Sociological Review*, vol. 33, pp. 20–30.

McCarthy, D. and Saegert, S. (1978), 'Residential density, social overload and social withdrawal', *Human Ecology*, vol. 6, no. 3, pp. 253–72.

Macaulay, J. and Berkowitz, L. (1970), *Altruism and Helping Behavior* (New York: Academic Press).

McKinlay, J. B. (1973), 'Social networks, lay consultation and help-seeking behaviour', *Social Forces*, vol. 51, no. 3, March, pp. 275–91.

Maguire, L. (1983), *Understanding Social Networks* (Beverly Hills: Sage).

Malinowski, B. (1922), *Argonauts of the Western Pacific: an account of native enterprise and adventure in the archipelagoes of Melanesian New Guinea* (London: Routledge & Kegan Paul).

Malson, M. (1982), 'The social support systems of black families', *Marriage and Family Review*, vol. 5, no. 4, winter, pp. 37–57.

Marshall, G., Rose, D., Vogler, C. and Newby, H. (1985), 'Class, citizenship and distributional conflict in modern Britain', *British Journal of Sociology*, vol. 36, no. 2, pp. 259–84.

Mauss, M. (1925), 'Essai sur le don: forme et raison de l'échange dans les sociétés archaiques', *L'Année Sociologique* n.s., vol. 1, pp. 30–186; translated by I. G. Cunnison as M. Mauss, *The Gift: forms and functions of exchange in archaic societies* (London: Cohen & West, 1966).

Mayer, P. (1961), *Tribesmen or Townsmen: Conservatism and the Process of Urbanization in a South African City* (Cape Town: Oxford University Press).

Mitchell, J. C. (1966), 'Theoretical orientations in African urban studies', in M. Banton (ed.), *The Social Anthropology of Complex Societies* (London: Tavistock), pp. 37–68.

Mitchell, J. C. (1969), 'The concept and use of social networks' in J. C. Mitchell (ed.), *Social Networks in Urban Situations* (Manchester: Manchester University Press), pp. 1–50.

Mogey, J. M. (1956), *Family and Neighbourhood* (Oxford: Oxford University Press).

Morris, D. and Hess, K. (1975), *Neighbourhood Power: the new localism* (Boston: Beacon Press).

Mount, F. (1982), *The Subversive Family: an alternative history of love and marriage* (London: Cape).

Muir, W. K. (1977), *Police: Street Corner Politicians* (Chicago: University of Chicago Press).

Naegale, K. (1958), 'Friendship and acquaintances: an exploration of some social distinctions', *Harvard Educational Review*, vol. 28, pp. 232–52.

National Commission on Neighborhoods (1979), *People, Building Neighborhoods* (Final Report to the President and Congress) (Washington, DC: US Government Printing Office).

Nelson, J. I. (1966), 'Clique contacts and family orientations'. *American Sociological Review*, vol. 31, no. 5, pp. 663–72.

Newby, H., Vogler, C., Rose, D. and Marshall, G. (1985), 'From Class Structure to Class Action: British working class politics in the 1980s', in B. Roberts *et al.* (eds.), *New Approaches to Economic Life* (Manchester: Manchester University Press), pp. 86–102.

Nisbet, R. (1966), *The Sociological Tradition* (New York: Basic Books).

Noddings, N. (1984), *Caring: a feminine approach to ethics and moral education* (Berkeley, Calif.: University of California Press).

Nuckolls, K. *et al.* (1982), 'Psychosocial assets, life crisis and the prognosis of pregnancy', *American Journal of Epidemiology*, vol. 95, pp. 431–41.

Offer, J. (1984), 'Informal Welfare, Social Work and the Sociology of Welfare', *British Journal of Social Work*, vol. 14, pp. 545–55.

Pahl, R. E. (1966), 'The rural–urban continuum', *Sociologia Ruralis*, vol. 6, no. 3–4, pp. 299–329.

Pahl, R. E. (1984), *Divisions of Labour* (Oxford: Blackwell).

Paine, R. (1967), 'What is gossip about? an alternative hypothesis', *Man* n.s. 2, pp. 278–85.

Pancoast, D. L., Parker, P. and Froland, C. (eds.) (1983), *Rediscovering Self-Help: its role in social care* (Beverly Hills: Sage).

Parker, G. (1985), *With Due Care and Attention: a review of research on informal care* (London: Family Policy Studies Centre).

Parker, R. (1981), 'Tending and social policy', in E. M. Goldberg and S. Hatch (eds.), *A New Look at the Personal Social Services* (London: Policy Studies Institute Discussion Paper no. 4), pp. 17–34.

Pember-Reeves, M. S. (1913), *Round About a Pound a Week* (London: Bell).

Peplau, L. A. and Perlman, D. (eds.) (1982), *Loneliness: a sourcebook of current theory, research and therapy* (New York: Wiley).

Pfiel, E. (1968), 'The pattern of neighbourhood relations in Dortmund-Neustadt' in R. E. Pahl (ed.), *Readings in Urban Sociology* (Oxford: Pergamon), pp. 135–58.

Pilisuk, M. and Minkler, M. (1985), 'Social support: economic and political considerations', *Social Policy* vol. 16, no. 3, winter, pp. 6–11.

Pilisuk, M. and Parks, S. H. (1986), *The Healing Web: Social Networks and Human Survival* (Hanover, N.H. University of New England Press).

Pinker, R. (1979), *The Idea of Welfare* (London: Heinemann).

Pinker, R. (1985), 'Social Policy and Social Care: Divisions of Responsibility', in J. A. Yoder *et al.* (eds.), *Support Networks in a Caring Community* (Dordrecht: Martinus Nijhoff), pp. 103–21.

Pitt-Rivers, J. (1973), 'The kith and the kin', in J. Goody (ed.), *The Character of Kinship* (Cambridge: Cambridge University Press), pp. 89–105.

Plant, R., Lesser, H. and Taylor-Gooby, P. (1980), *Political Philosophy and Social Welfare: essays on the normative basis of welfare provision* (London: Routledge & Kegan Paul).

Poggi, G. (1972), *Images of Society: essays on the sociological theories of Tocqueville, Marx and Durkheim* (Stanford: Stanford University Press).

Polanyi, K. (1957), 'The economy as an instituted process', in K. Polanyi, C. M. Arensberg and H. W. Pearson (eds.), *Trade and Market in the Early Empires: Economies in History and Theory* (Glencoe, Ill.: Free Press), pp. 243–70.

Price, F. V. (1981), 'Only connect? issues in charting social networks', *Sociological Review*, vol. 29, no. 2, pp. 283–312.

Pruger, R. (1973), 'Social policy: unilateral transfer or reciprocal exchange', *Journal of Social Policy*, vol. 2, no. 4, pp. 289–302.

Qureshi, H. (1985), 'Exchange theory and helpers on the Kent Community Care Scheme', *Research, Policy and Planning*, vol. 3, no. 1, pp. 1–9.

Qureshi, H., Challis, D. and Davies, B. (1983), 'Motivations and rewards for helpers in the Kent Community Care Scheme', in Hatch (ed.) (1983), pp. 144–68.

Qureshi, H., Davies, B. and Challis, D. (1979), 'Motivations and rewards of volunteers and informal care givers', *Journal of Voluntary Action Research*, vol. 8, nos. 1–2, pp. 47–55.

Radcliffe-Brown, A. R. (1940), 'On social structure', *Journal of the Royal Anthropological Institute of Great Britain and Ireland*, vol. 70, pp. 1–12.

Rainwater, L. (1966), 'Crucible of identity: the negro lower-class family', *Daedalus*, vol. 95, no. 2, pp. 172–216.

Rainwater, L. and Yancey, W. (eds.) (1967), *The Moynihan Report and the Politics of Controversy* (Cambridge, Mass.: MIT).

Richardson, A. and Goodman, M. (1983), *Self-Help and Social Care: mutual aid organisations in practice* (London: Policy Studies Institute Report no. 612).

Roberts, R. (1973), *The Classic Slum: Salford Life in the First Quarter of the Century* (Harmondsworth: Penguin).

Roberts, R. (1978), *A Ragged Schooling: growing up in the classic slum* (London: Fontana).

Robinson, F. and Abrams, P. (1977), *What We Know About The Neighbours: A Working Paper* (University of Durham: Rowntree Research Unit, mimeo).

Robinson, F. and Robinson, S. (1981), *Neighbourhood Care: An Exploratory Bibliography* (Berkhamsted, Hertfordshire: The Volunteer Centre).

Roethlisberger, F. J. and Dickson, W. J. (1939), *Management and the Worker: Technical v. Social Organisation in an Industrial Plant* (Cambridge, Mass.: Harvard University Press).

Rose, H. (1974), 'Up Against the Welfare State: The Claimants' Unions', in R. Miliband and J. Saville (eds.), *The Socialist Register 1973* (London: Merlin Press), pp. 179–203.

Rosnow, R. L. and Fine, G. A. (1976), *Rumor and Gossip: the social psychology of hearsay* (New York: Elsevier).

Ross, E. (1983), 'Survival Networks: women's neighbourhood sharing in London before World War 1', *History Workshop Journal*, vol. 15, spring, pp. 4–27.

Rosser, C. and Harris, C. C. (1965), *The Family and Social Change* (London: Routledge & Kegan Paul).

Rossi, A. S. (1984), 'Gender and Parenthood', *American Sociological Review*, vol. 49, pp. 1–19.

Rossiter, C. and Wicks, M. (1982), *Crisis or Challenge: Family Care,*

Elderly People and Social Policy (London: Study Commission on the Family).

Rothman, J. and Warren, D. I. (1981), 'Community networks', in M. E. Olsen and M. Micklin (eds.), *Handbook of Applied Sociology: frontiers of contemporary research* (New York: Praeger), pp. 134–56.

Royal Commission on Mental Illness and Mental Deficiency (1957), *Report* (Cmnd. 169) (London: HMSO).

Rule, J. (1973), *Private Lives and Public Surveillance* (London: Allen Lane).

Rushton, J. P. and Sorrentino, R. M. (eds.) (1981), *Altruism and Helping Behavior: Social, Personality and Developmental Perspectives* (Hillsdale, NJ: L. Erlbaum Associates).

Sahlins, M. D. (1965), 'On the sociology of primitive exchange', in M. Banton (ed.), *The Relevance of Models for Social Anthropology* (London: Tavistock), pp. 139–236.

Sainsbury, P. and De Alarçon, J. (1974), 'The Cost of Community Care and the Burden on the Family of Treating the Mentally Ill at Home', in D. Lees and S. Shaw (eds.), *Impairment, Disability and Handicap* (London: Heinemann Educational), pp. 123–40.

Schmalenbach, H. (1961), 'The sociological category of communion', in T. Parsons, E. Shils, K. D. Naegale and J. R. Pitts (eds.), *Theories of Society*, vol. I (Glencoe, Ill.: Free Press), pp. 331–47.

Seebohm Report (1968), *Report of the Committee on Local Authority and Allied Personal Social Services* (Cmnd. 3703) (London: HMSO).

Sennett, R. (1970), *Families Against the City: Middle Class Homes of Industrial Chicago 1872-90* (Cambridge, Mass.: Harvard University Press).

Shanas, E., Townsend, P., Wedderburn, D., Friis, N., Milhøj, P. and Stenhouwer, J. (1968), *Old People in Three Industrial Societies* (London: Routledge & Kegan Paul).

Sharpe, L. J. (1975), 'The social scientist and policy-making', *Policy and Politics*, vol. 4, no. 2, pp. 7–34 (partially reprinted in Bulmer (ed.), 1978, pp. 302–12).

Sharpe, L. J. and Newton, K. (1984), *Does Politics Matter? the determinants of public policy* (Oxford: Clarendon Press).

Sheldon, J. H. (1948), *The Social Medicine of Old Age* (London: Oxford University Press).

Scottish Home and Health Department (1980), *Changing Patterns of Care* (Advisory Council on Social Work and Scottish Health Service Planning Council (Scottish Home and Health Department, Edinburgh)) (London: HMSO).

Shils, E. (1951), 'The Study of the Primary Group', in D. Lerner and H. D. Lasswell (eds.), *The Policy Sciences: recent developments in scope and method* (Stanford, Calif.: Stanford University Press), pp. 44–69.

Shils, E. (1957), 'Primordial, Personal, Sacred and Civil Ties: some particular observations on the relationships of sociological theory and research', *British Journal of Sociology*, vol. 8, pp. 130–45.

Shils, E. and Janowitz, M. (1948), 'Cohesion and disintegration in the *Wehrmacht*', *Public Opinion Quarterly*, vol. 12, pp. 280–315.

Shulman, N. (1967), 'Mutual aid and neighboring patterns', *Anthropologica*, vol. 9, pp. 51–60.

Shulman, N. (1976), 'Network analysis: a new addition to an old bag of tricks', *Acta Sociologica*, vol. 19, no. 4, pp. 307–23.

Simmel, G. (1950), 'The Metropolis and Mental Life', in K. Wolff (translator and editor), *The Sociology of Georg Simmel* (New York: The Free Press), pp. 409–24.

Singer, P. (1983), 'The blood feud: round two', *Hastings Center Report*, vol. 13, no. 4, August, pp. 48–50.

Slater, P. (1970), *The Pursuit of Loneliness: American culture at the breaking point* (Boston: Beacon Press).

Smith, T. S. (1985), 'Personal ties and institutional action: an aggregate analysis of rates of reciprocated choice in friendship markets', in Suttles and Zald (eds.) (1985), pp. 23–51.

Sorokin, P. A. (1950), *Altruistic Love: a study of American Good Neighbours and Christian Saints* (Boston: Beacon Press).

Specht, H. (1986), 'Social support, social networks, social exchange and social work practice', *Social Service Review*, vol. 60, no. 2, pp. 218–40.

Stacey, M. (1969), 'The myth of community studies', *British Journal of Sociology*, vol. 20, no. 2, pp. 134–47.

Stack, C. (1974), *All Our Kin: Strategies for Survival in a Black Community* (New York: Harper & Row).

Stevenson, O. (1980), *The Realities of A Caring Community* (Eleanor Rathbone Memorial Lecture, University of Liverpool).

Stouffer, S. A. *et al.* (1949), *The American Soldier* (Princeton, NJ: Princeton University Press).

Sugden, R. (1984), 'Reciprocity: the supply of public goods through voluntary contributions', *Economic Journal*, vol. 94, December, pp. 772–87.

Susser, I. (1982), *Norman Street: Poverty and Politics in an Urban Neighborhood* (New York: Oxford University Press).

Sussman, M. B. (1977), 'Family, bureaucracy and the elderly individual: an organisational linkage perspective', in E. Shanas and M. B. Sussman (eds.), *Family, Bureaucracy and the Elderly* (Durham, NC: Duke University Press), pp. 2–20.

Suttles, G. D. (1968), *The Social Order of the Slum* (Chicago: University of Chicago Press).

Suttles, G. D. (1970), 'Friendship as a social institution', in G. J. McCall *et al.*, *Social Relationships* (Chicago: Aldine), pp. 95–135.

Suttles, G. D. and Zald, M. N. (eds.) (1985), *The Challenge of Social Control: Citizenship and Institution Building in Modern Society: Essays in Honor of Morris Janowitz* (Norwood, NJ: Ablex).

Thoits, P. (1982), 'Conceptual, methodological and theoretical problems in studying social support as a buffer against life stress', *Journal of Health and Social Behavior*, vol. 21, pp. 145–59.

Thomas, D. N. (1985), 'Private Lives', *Community Care*, 7 February, pp. 16–18.

Thomas, D. N. (1986), *White Bolts, Black Locks: participation in the inner city* (London: Allen & Unwin).

Thrasher, F. (1928), *The Gang* (Chicago: University of Chicago Press).

Titmuss, R. M. (1968), 'Community care: fact or fiction', in R. Titmuss, *Commitment to Welfare* (London: George Allen & Unwin), pp. 104–09.

Titmuss, R. M. (1970), *The Gift Relationship: from human blood to social policy* (London: Allen & Unwin).

Toennies, F. (1957), *Community and Society (Gemeinschaft und Gesellschaft)* (translated and edited by C. P. Loomis) (East Lansing, Michigan: Michigan State University Press).

Tornstam, L. (1981), 'Daily problems in various ages', Paper presented to 12th International Congress of Gerontology, Hamburg, 11–17 July.

Townsend, P. (1963), *The Family Life of Old People* (Harmondsworth: Penguin) (first published 1957).

Townsend, P. and Tunstall, S. (1973), 'Sociological explanations of the lonely', in Peter Townsend, *The Social Minority* (London: Allen Lane), pp. 240–66.

Tunstall, J. (1968), *Old and Alone* (London: Routledge & Kegan Paul).

Ungerson, C. (1983a), 'Why do women care?' in J. Finch and D. Groves (eds.), *A Labour of Love* (London: Routledge & Kegan Paul), pp. 31–49.

Ungerson, C. (1983b), 'Women and caring: skills, tasks and taboos', in Gamarnikov *et al.* (1983), pp. 62–77.

Ungerson, C. (1987), *Nursing for Nothing* (London: Tavistock).

Urmson, J. O. (1969), 'Saints and heroes', in J. Fineberg (ed.), *Moral Concepts* (Oxford: Oxford University Press).

Uttley, S. (1980), 'The welfare exchange reconsidered', *Journal of Social Policy*, vol. 9, no. 2, pp. 187–206.

Walker, A. (ed.) (1982), *Community Care: The Family, the State and Social Policy* (Oxford: Basil Blackwell and Martin Robertson).

Walker, A. (1986), 'Community Care: Fact and Fiction', in P. Willmott (ed.) (1986), pp. 4–15.

Wallace, C. (1984), 'Informal Work in Two Neighbourhoods: Warden Bay and Rushenden' (Canterbury: University of Kent, Work Behaviour Research Unit, mimeo).

Wallace, C. and Pahl, R. E. (1984), 'Polarisation, unemployment and all forms of work' (Canterbury: University of Kent Work Behaviour Research Unit, mimeo).

Walzer, M. (1981), 'The distribution of membership', in P. G. Brown and H. Shue (eds.), *Boundaries: national autonomy and its limits* (Totowa, NJ: Rowman and Littlefield), pp. 1–35.

Warner, W. L. and Lunt, P. S. (1941), *The Social Life of a Modern Community* (New Haven, Conn.: Yale University Press).

Watson, D. (1985), *A Code of Ethics for Social Work: the second step* (London: Routledge & Kegan Paul).

Weale, A. (1978), *Equality and Social Policy* (London: Routledge & Kegan Paul).

Webb, A. and Wistow, G. (1982), 'The personal social services: incrementalism, expediency or systematic social planning', in A. Walker (ed.), *Public Expenditure and Social Policy* (London: Heinemann), pp. 137–64.

Weber, M. (1947), *The Theory of Social and Economic Organisation* (ed. T. Parsons) (New York: Oxford University Press).

Weiner, F. H. (1976), 'Altruism, ambiance and action: the effect of rural and urban rearing on helping behavior', *Journal of Personality and Social Psychology*, vol. 34, no. 1, pp. 112–24.

Weiss, R. S. (1969), 'The fund of sociability', *Trans-action/Society*, vol. 6, no. 9, pp. 36–43.

Weiss, R. S. (1973a), *Loneliness: the experience of emotional and social isolation* (Cambridge, Mass.: MIT Press).

Weiss, R. S. (1973b), 'Helping relationships: relationships of clients with physicians, social workers, priests and others', *Social Problems*, vol. 20, no. 3, pp. 319–29.

Weiss, R. S. (1975), 'The provisions of social relationships', in Z. Rubin (ed.), *Doing Unto Others* (Englewood Cliffs, NJ: Prentice Hall), pp. 47–72.

Weiss, R. S. (1976), 'Transition states and other stressful situations: their nature and programs for their management', in G. Caplan and M. Killilea (eds.), *Support Systems & Mutual Help: multidisciplinary explorations* (New York: Grune & Stratton), pp. 213–32.

Weiss, R. S. (1982), 'Issues in the study of loneliness', in Peplau and Perlman (1982), pp. 71–80.

Wellman, B. (1979), 'The community question: the intimate networks of East Yorkers', *American Journal of Sociology*, vol. 84, no. 5, pp. 1201–31.

Wellman, B. (1981), 'Applying network analysis to the study of support', in Gottleib (ed.) (1981), pp. 171–200.

Wellman, B. (1983), 'Network analysis: some basic principles', in R. Collins (ed.), *Sociological Theory 1983* (San Francisco: Jossey Bass), pp. 155–200.

Wellman, B. and Hiscott, R. (1985), 'From social support to social network', in I. Sarason and B. Sarason (eds.), *Social Support: Theory, Research, Applications* (Dordrecht: Martinus Nijhoff), pp. 205–222.

Wellman, B. and Leighton, B. (1979), 'Networks, neighbourhoods and communities: approaches to the study of the community question', *Urban Affairs Quarterly*, vol. 14, no. 3, March, pp. 363–90.

Wenger, G. C. (1981), *The Elderly in the Community: family contacts, social integration and community involvement* (University College of North Wales, Bangor, Department of Social Theory and Institutions, Working Paper 18, mimeo).

Wenger, G. C. (1982), 'Ageing in rural communities: family contacts and community integration', *Ageing and Society*, vol. 2, no. 2, pp. 211–29.

Wenger, G. C. (1983), 'Loneliness: a problem of measurement', in D. Jerrome (ed.), *Ageing in Modern Society: contemporary approaches* (London: Croom Helm), pp. 145–67.

Wenger, G. C. (1984), *The Supportive Network: coping with old age* (London: Allen & Unwin).

West, P., Illsley, R. and Kelman, H. (1984), 'Public preferences for the care of dependency groups', *Social Science and Medicine* 18, pp. 287–95.

Westin, A. F. (1970), *Privacy and Freedom* (London: Bodley Head).

White, J. (1986), *The Worst Street in North London: Campbell Bunk, Islington Between the Wars* (London: Routledge & Kegan Paul).

Whittaker, J. K. (1983), 'Mutual helping in human service practice', in J. K. Whittaker and J. Garbarino (eds.), *Social Support Networks: Informal Helping in the Human Services* (New York: Aldine), pp. 33–67.

Wiebe, R. (1967), *The Search for Order 1877–1920* (New York: Hill & Wang).

Wilcox, B. J. (1981), 'Social support in adjusting to marital disruption: a network analysis', in Gottleib (ed.) (1981), pp. 97–115.

Williams, B. (1973), *Morality* (Harmondsworth: Penguin).

Williams, R. (1973), *The Country and the City* (London: Chatto & Windus).

Williams, R. (1976), *Keywords* (London: Fontana).

Willmott, P. (with D. Thomas) (1984), *Community in Social Policy* (Discussion Paper no. 9) (London: Policy Studies Institute).

Willmott, P. (1986a), *Social Networks, Informal Care and Public Policy* (London: Policy Studies Institute Research Report no. 655).

Willmott, P. (ed.) (1986b), *The Debate About Community: Papers from a seminar on 'Community and Social Policy'* (London: Policy Studies Institute Discussion Paper no. 13).

Willmott, P. (1987), *Friendship Networks and Social Support: a study in a London suburb* (London: Policy Studies Institute).

Willmott, Phyllis (1984), 'Helping in other people's homes', *Self Health* no. 4, September, pp. 22–3.

Wilson, E. (1982), 'Women, the "Community" and the "Family"', in A. Walker (ed.) (1982), pp. 40–55.

Wilson, S. J. (1978), *Confidentiality in Social Work: issues and principles* (New York: Free Press).

Wirth, L. (1938), 'Urbanism as a way of life', *American Journal of Sociology*, vol. 44, pp. 3–24.

Wolfe, A. W. (1978), 'The rise of network thinking in anthropology', *Social Networks*, vol. 1, pp. 53–64.

Yoder, J. A., Jonker, J. M. L. and Leaper, R. A. B. (eds.) (1985), *Social Networks in a Caring Community* (Dordrecht: Martinus Nijhoff).

Young, M. and Willmott, P. (1957, 1962), *Family and Kinship in East London* (London: Routledge & Kegan Paul and Harmondsworth: Penguin) (New edition with new introduction, London: Routledge & Kegan Paul, 1986).

Young, M. and Willmott, P. (1975), *The Symmetrical Family: a study of work and leisure in the London region* (Harmondsworth: Penguin).

Zito, J. M. (1974), 'Anonymity and neighbouring in an urban, high-rise complex', *Urban Life and Culture*, vol. 3, no. 3, pp. 243–63.

Index